BECOMING A
DOCTOR

From Student to Specialist,
Doctor-Writers Share Their Experiences

Edited by LEE GUTKIND

W. W. NORTON & COMPANY
NEW YORK ■ LONDON

Copyright © 2010 by Creative Nonfiction Foundation
Introduction copyright © 2010 by Lee Gutkind

For information about permission to reproduce selections from
this book, write to Permissions, W. W. Norton & Company, Inc.,
500 Fifth Avenue, New York, NY 10110

For information about special discounts for bulk purchases, please contact
W. W. Norton Special Sales at specialsales@wwnorton.com or 800-233-4830

Manufacturing by Courier Westford
Book design by Ellen Cipriano
Production manager: Julia Druskin

Library of Congress Cataloging-in-Publication Data

Becoming a doctor : from student to specialist : doctor-writers share
their experiences / edited by Lee Gutkind. — 1st ed.
p. ; cm.
Includes bibliographical references.
ISBN 978-0-393-07156-6 (hardcover)
1. Physicians' writings. I. Gutkind, Lee. [DNLM:
1. Physicians—psychology. 2. Education, Medical.
3. Medicine. 4. Personal Narratives. W 21 B3975 2010]
R134.B43 2010
610.92—dc22

                                        2009040428

ISBN 978-0-393-33455-5 pbk.

W. W. Norton & Company, Inc.
500 Fifth Avenue, New York, N.Y. 10110
www.wwnorton.com

W. W. Norton & Company Ltd.
Castle House, 75/76 Wells Street, London W1T 3QT

1 2 3 4 5 6 7 8 9 0

More Praise for *Becoming a Doctor*

"First-rate writers. . . . The essayists in Gutkind's book are good people not because they are distinguished doctors and writers; instead, the quality of their medical practice as well as their art extends from their acute ability to empathize with others."

—Linda Elisabeth Beattie, *Courier-Journal*

"The book humanizes the figure in the lab coat."

—Rachel Saslow, *Washington Post*

"Medical students and medical professionals will enjoy these perspectives on their profession; they will likely encounter or have encountered many of the obstacles narrated."

—Dana Ladd, *Library Journal*

"Through honest and beautiful writing, these physicians reveal themselves as caregivers and as people—sometimes courageous, often imperfect, and always deeply, deeply human."

—Vincent Lam, MD, author of the Giller Prize–winning *Bloodletting and Miraculous Cures*

"Here, some of the best-known names in medical writing are joined by powerful new voices to help elucidate the mysterious and grueling transformation from non-doctor to doctor. . . . A remarkable collection."   —Christine Montross, MD, author of *Body of Work: Meditations on Mortality from the Human Anatomy Lab*

"[S]tunningly honest stories. . . . You will find no saints or superheroes here: just humans who struggle daily to balance competence and compassion."   —Paul Austin, MD, author of *Something for the Pain*

"Readers of this collection of stories, dramas, tableaux, still lives, dreams, laments, and obituaries undergo in imagination the sorrow, the fear, and the awe of every doctor. The texts stand as a testimony to medicine's resonance and reality."   —Rita Charon, MD, PhD, director, Program in Narrative Medicine, Columbia University

ALSO EDITED BY LEE GUTKIND

CONTENTS

Contents

INTRODUCTION:
WRITING ABOUT DOCTORS

Lee Gutkind

So far in my career I have written four books about doctors—organ transplant surgeons, pediatricians, child psychiatrists, and veterinarians—and their patients. I have also written books about backwoodsmen, roboticists, baseball umpires, and other subjects, all compelling and interesting and provocative, but always I come back to medicine.

There are some obvious reasons for a writer to find endless fascination with doctors and their lives, especially a writer of creative nonfiction, the genre that makes fact more compelling and understandable through narrative. For one thing, the practice of medicine, especially in a high-acuity medical center (though also in private practice), is exciting and dramatic; there are plenty of stories to capture and relate. Every day brings new narratives and scenes populated by colorful and controversial characters, real people and their loved ones, who are often in real trouble. The raw material couldn't be more exciting, mysterious, and obviously—for better or worse—life-changing.

Throughout many years of shadowing doctors as they work, I've seen patients rolled into the operating room on the absolute edge of death, then pacing the hospital corridor a week later, ready and anxious for discharge and home. I have seen patients die in the operating room, and physicians weeping in helpless frustration, although, thankfully, failure is not as frequent as success. I've seen patients terrified and confused because no one can understand what is wrong with them, why they feel so poorly or so frightened, until the right specialist—or therapist—somehow, magically, translates their symptoms into a diagnosis or quells their anxiety with assurance.

It's not magic, of course. Success in medicine stems from a combination of clear thinking, hard work, repeated practice, and old-fashioned grit—often with many mistakes and false starts along the way. I would describe the writing process in the same way. Talent is important, but not necessarily the key component. Effective, powerful writing, like effective doctoring, demands a rare ability to avoid becoming discouraged while experiencing frustration—and the willingness, energy, and fortitude to keep trying. Ernest Hemingway frequently pointed out that he wrote the last chapter of A Farewell to Arms thirty-nine times, until he got it right. The best doctors and the best writers live and breathe this "never give up, never give in" philosophy.

In addition to possessing grit and determination, doctors, like nonfiction writers, learn to think analytically, unraveling and reconstructing the intimate details of a patient's story from beginning to end. The doctor has to understand and solve the narrative quickly, just like a writer, although the writer writes a story to keep a reader engaged, while the doctor wants to find fast relief for his or her patient. (And these days, quick, efficient, effective work by the physician is mandated by managed care.)

Writers and doctors also share an intensity of obsession. Their hours are sporadic and often overwhelming, dictated by need rather than plans and schedules. While private practice may sometimes be less demanding than working in the trenches of a medical center, doctors' personal lives are invariably determined by events beyond their control.

Writing about doctors has helped me to realize that they aren't necessarily special people; they are, more precisely, ordinary people engaged in an extraordinary profession. Clearly, they are not perfect—not as doctors or as people. Sometimes doctors are distant and convey disinterest; sometimes they are egocentric and radiate superiority; sometimes they are angry or frustrated and treat people rudely; sometimes, alas, the health care system makes it impossible for them to do their jobs—and to demonstrate passion and empathy for their patients and colleagues when they most want to. The responsibilities of doctoring often surprise, test, and challenge them—but the best doctors meet and, when necessary, exceed the challenges. And the truth is, we ask more of our doctors, especially these days, than we do of people in almost any other profession.

Most of the doctors I have met—and there have been a great many over the years—have had a great appreciation for literature. And while relatively few of the doctors I have known had any urge to be creative writers, doctors who do write often show a real talent for telling stories and communicating complicated information in layman's terms. Perhaps this has to do with their growing awareness of the need to understand their patients' stories in order to understand how to treat them, and the importance of communicating so that their patients understand their message.

When doctors do sit down to write, they have a wealth of experiences and raw material to draw on. Physicians' professional lives are steeped in drama; health and sickness, life and death, fear and courage, clarity and confusion are part of their daily routine. The fact that the stakes are so high in almost everything they do, in training or practice, leads to daily exhilaration and anxiety, but also to the need for personal analysis and reflection and an ability to roll with the punches, as the essays in this collection demonstrate.

In these pages, Perri Klass, a pediatrician, explains why she insists that her students appreciate the unique opportunity to learn from their patients' stories as well as their bodies. Elissa Ely humbly accepts that the road to stability for one of her psychiatric patients requires that she, the doctor, follow instead of lead. Sandeep Jauhar discovers that a physician's words can occasionally do as much damage as good. Sayantani DasGupta vividly portrays the driven mania of an intern. Chris Stookey tells the story of being hit with a mysterious malpractice suit as a resident. Lauren Slater probes the tragic ambivalence she feels about having walked away from her profession. And Robert Coles looks back on his intimate and inspiring relationship with the poet William Carlos Williams.

In this book about writers who are doctors and doctors who are writers, the two professions come together. After all, doctors are always writing patient and professional scenarios in their heads, rejoicing in their successes and reliving the ways in which they feel they were ineffective—or worse. What doctors do—everything they do—goes far beyond the act or the service itself. Their decisions and actions affect many people they will never know; in this way they are just like writers, whose books and essays, once written, take on a life of their own and affect readers in unknown and unpredictable ways. Perhaps, in the end, this is why so many doctors write: in their writing, not only their words and ideas but the people they write about will always live, if only on paper.

ACKNOWLEDGMENTS

This book was inspired by Karen Wolk Feinstein, president and CEO of the Jewish Healthcare Foundation. Dedicated to supporting health care services, education, and research to encourage medical advancement and protect vulnerable populations, the JHF has generously supported this and other projects, working with me and *Creative Nonfiction*, the magazine I edit, in the form not only of grants but also of friendship and encouragement.

Becoming a Doctor is the first in a new series of medical narrative books supported by the JHF. I hope that the essays collected here help demonstrate the awesome challenges and frustrations facing the medical community, especially doctors, who must too often fight systems that impede patient care. More than that, I hope this book is a valuable addition to the health care debate in this country, and that the stories collected here might have an impact, and help bring about changes that are needed if not just any of us, but all of us, are to receive quality care.

Acknowledgments

This book is a product of Dr. Feinstein's vision, which, along with support from the foundation she leads, made my work as editor and the work of the writers in this book possible. On behalf of the writers and staff at *Creative Nonfiction* who worked on *Becoming a Doctor*, I would like to thank Karen Wolk Feinstein and her colleagues at the Jewish Healthcare Foundation—particularly Nancy Zionts and Carla Barricella—not only for their insight, inspiration, and support but also for their faith in the power of true stories and bold voices.

I would also like to thank attorney Melissa Irr Harkes for her thorough and conscientious legal vetting and writer/editor Donna Hogarty for fact-checking this manuscript; Amy Cherry, our editor at W. W. Norton, and Andrew Blauner, our longtime agent and friend, for their wisdom and support; the Juliet Lea Hillman Simonds Foundation and the Pennsylvania Council on the Arts, whose ongoing support has been essential to the Creative Nonfiction Foundation's success; and Hattie Fletcher, managing editor of *Creative Nonfiction*, who is a skillful editor and eminently reliable sounding board, and the glue that keeps CNF together.

Last but not least, Stephen Knezovich, associate editor of *Creative Nonfiction*, worked closely with me and with all of the writers from the very beginning of this project, providing regular communication, feedback, advice, and solid editorial counsel. His contribution has been invaluable.

DISCLAIMER

Some names and identifying details have been changed to protect the identities of people and institutions mentioned in these essays.

INTERN

Sayantani DasGupta

She hoarded index cards and Xeroxed protocols and carefully transcribed antibiotic dosing regimens. She hoarded miniaturized growth charts and lists of developmental milestones and near-pornographic images of breast and genital development at various Tanner stages. She hoarded code cards, an instruction sheet on intubation, and a much creased flowchart on diabetic ketoacidosis ripped out of a textbook. She hoarded her Harriet Lane handbook—the most important pages falling out and held in place by a large purple rubber band.

She hoarded the calculator that hung around her neck on an uncomfortable metal chain along with her ID and electronic pass card. She hoarded tongue depressors, folded-up paper measuring tape, gauze pads, and gauze rolls. She hoarded IVs, packaged tubing connectors, and an occasional infant's arm board. She hoarded plastic ear cleaners and long, clear tubes full of black otoscope specula. She hoarded individually wrapped packets of alcohol—which she used for wiping her stethoscope, as well as getting blood off her jacket or shoes. She hoarded rolls of tape—the plastic kind, not the cloth—and the immensely useful little butterfly adhesive strips.

She hoarded rubber tourniquets—one strung through her button-holes she was willing to share and a backup stashed in her top pocket she was not. She hoarded the beautiful packets of butterfly needles—her favorite light blue 21 gauge and second favorite indigo 23 gauge and one or two of the obscenely large 19 gauge which she saved for the adolescents.

She hoarded guaiac development cards, six or seven at a time. She hoarded the bottles of chemical developer with their yellow screw-on tops to test the stool for blood once smeared on the card. These were precious on the floor, impossible to find when you needed them, so she hoarded them, risking the telltale astringent leak in the bottom of her pocket. She hoarded all this because there was nothing worse than standing in a patient's room with a gloved finger full of excrement and nowhere to put it.

She hoarded all the free drug company stuff. (Screw the ethics.) A squeaky duck to hang on her stethoscope, a notepad shaped like a fire truck, a cardboard wheel to help her calculate a teenager's weeks of gestation based on her last menstrual period. And of course, she hoarded the pens. The pens from Advair and Amoxil, from Zithromax and Zyrtec. She hoarded pens from Ventolin and even ones from Viagra, which were so comfortingly heavy in her hand and, understandably, rare on the pediatric floors.

She hoarded her patients—especially the usually healthy infants admitted to "rule out sepsis." Those chubby babies were as close to entirely well as one could get in the hospital. She hoarded their piglet toes, their ham-hock thighs. She hoarded their round cheeks and buttocks, their jiggly bellies hanging thickly over diapers like ripe melons or pop 'n' fresh biscuits. She hoarded their thick fingers, their curving ears, their trufflelike noses. She hoarded the feeling of them, calm and warm against her chest. Sometimes, during a hard night on call, she escaped to the infants' floor just to hold and rock a baby. When she felt the weight of their bodies against hers, she hoarded the ache somewhere below the pit of her stomach.

She hoarded her body and its senses—taste, primarily, because she found herself so empty. She hoarded memories of meals, rolling the recalled tastes around and around her mouth like marbles—creamy homemade soups, fluffy omelets, shrimp curry made with gigantic prawns. At the hospital, it was all sugary donuts during morning report, tepid pizza during noon conference, an occasional catered lecture with dry turkey on even drier rye bread. The coffee, which she drank in excess, was always dark and dingy in Styrofoam cups that made her teeth ache. She hoarded the desire for a cup of perfectly brewed Darjeeling tea, served in a china cup, like her now dead grandmother would have made it.

She missed the feeling of her own skin, and hoarded travel-size tubes of hand cream she bought on a near-daily basis from the hospital giftshop. The lotion in the patients' supply closet had to do when she couldn't spare the time, but it left her smelling like the supply closet, or, worse, like the patients, and its watery consistency did very little to ease her rough, sobbing hands. The process of applying the lotion was a ritual of repetition. Grabbing the tube from her right pocket, she would dab a mound of lotion in the center of her left palm, then rub the moisture into the other with a Lady Macbeth–like hand-wringing gesture; interlacing her fingers to distribute the lotion evenly, she finished by circularly massaging her dry cuticles, one by one by one.

Her face, in contrast, was oilier than one of her adolescent patients', and she hoarded hairbands in her pockets, purse, and car to keep her thick hair away from its inexplicably slick surface. In the procedure room, when she would be assigned the task of holding down a squirming child for an IV, or if she was struggling to find a fat infant's rubbery veins under the chief resident's critical eyes, she would often feel the oil and sweat pouring down from her hairline, trickling under her glasses, making everything hot and cloudy, like the surface of some misty alien planet.

She hoarded astringent, perfume, and deodorant, all of which she used in abundance, and to seemingly little effect. She took long, warm showers as soon as she got home, and soon used up those tiny floral soaps she had been hoarding for years. For her birthday, she asked specifically for a basket of them from one of those stores in the mall that specialized in giddy floral aromas and overflowing gift displays. But no matter how much she bathed, or how expensive her soap, her nose seemed filled with the smells of the hospital, the sick, and her own stale and sticky body. The only time she remembered ever being so disgusted by her own stink was during Gross Anatomy, when the cloy of Formalin seemed to glom onto her skin, under her nails, and in her very nostril hairs.

She did not hoard sight and sound but rather hid from them. The too bright fluorescent lights, everything stark and bare, the same at 7 a.m. as at 2 a.m. True, there were images of bears and butterflies on the walls, but their cartoonish faces were slightly menacing, like clowns with too red, too wide smiles (even as a little girl, she had never liked clowns). Sounds were worse: the incessant crying, the overhead paging and beeping, the shouting of angry mothers and nurses for all the things she had done wrong that day—the delayed orders for pain medication, the incorrectly taped (and now fallen out) IVs. Worse still was the sound of professional humiliation—"pimping" by senior residents or attendings who knew you didn't know and kept asking you anyway. Sometimes, she walked around with imaginary fingers in her ears so that mouths moved but no sounds came out. She hoarded that albeit artificial tranquillity.

She hoarded her comfortable clogs, her absorbent socks, and her Victoria's Secret cotton underwear. There was no purpose in frilly undergarments that might ride up under scrub pants during a tense trip to the ICU. Yet, there seemed to be undue anxiety on the part of her august institution lest she make a less practical choice of attire. In fact, the resident handbook had a bizarrely complex set of dress codes—such that men were discouraged from wearing their hair long, growing beards, wearing jeans or T-shirts. Women were chastened to avoid open toe shoes, skirts above the knee, and shirts unbuttoned below the "sternomanubrial junction." Women were to wear their V-neck scrubs turned to the back, no rings in excess of a wedding band, and no long nails or "creatively colorful" nail polish. Clearly, the hospital was distressed at the thought of a breast popping out during a code, or a lawsuit by someone poked in the eye with a rhinestoned nail or diamond ring. None of it seemed to apply to her anyway—half the time she didn't remember she was a woman. Her entire body was usually ensconced in a two sizes too big unisex white coat, with roll-upable sleeves and too big pockets for all the things she was hoarding.

She hoarded sex, or at least, her memories of sex. The actual experience was rare. In fact, most of the time, she resented sex, not just because of the sleep she lost (which she calculated down to the minute on the glowing red digital clock) but also for its newfound difficulties. Whereas sex had once been mellow and honey-smooth, the combination of sleeplessness and stress had morphed intimacy into a jabbing and fearsome experience—a spiky medieval mace in her nether regions. If only she had kept quiet, perhaps her husband would not have lost so much interest after a mere six months of marriage. Crying during intimacy, as it turned out, was not such a turn-on for men. Worse still, her traitorous body seemed to have a malicious sense of humor; despite all the pain, she often found herself yearning—aching—to be touched. So she hoarded her dusty recollections of physical pleasure. In fact, the memory of being wanted would creep up on her at the most unexpected of times: when running a blood gas to the lab, calling a surgical consult, being awakened to rewrite a Tylenol order for the twentieth time. It trickled, hot and shameful, through her brittle veins like some lugubrious IV medication. She hoarded the thought, "Here I am no one, but in another place, another time, I have been loved."

As a substitute for sex, she hoarded the few things from her former life that made her feel alive, like poetry and dangling earrings (also discouraged by the handbook). When they had first been dating, in medical school, her husband would leave her poems to find in unexpected places. In his almost illegible handwriting, he would copy verse by Shakespeare and Emerson, Neruda and Rumi onto yellow sticky notes and post them on the bathroom mirror, tuck them into the windshield of her car, or stick them in her pharmacology textbook. Now, she rediscovered these notes from the secret places such memories are kept. She folded them like mystical mantras whose meaning has been made secondary to their symbolic power, tucking one into each of her scrubs pockets before a long call night. The words were too beautiful to read all at once, so she hoarded them, slipping a sentence into her cheek, a metaphor behind her ear, and, as if afraid of getting mugged, a really vivid image into her sock.

In the predawn mornings, after she parked her car in the hospital lot, she would sit a moment or two in the steel safety of the machine. In that stillness, she allowed herself to consider—would he wait until the end of internship to leave her? For the rest of the day and night, there would be no more time for such thoughts, but she made this small gesture in the mornings. Then she reminded herself that at least she would return, at some point in the near future, to that very spot behind the wheel. That she would be physically intact and that she would return. She hoarded the thought.

She hoarded her youth and her adulthood both at the same time. The former protected her from becoming one of the ancient adult patients she passed in the elevators and hallways, the ones with open, gangrenous footsores and half-missing upper jaws. The latter protected her from being one of the bald chemo kids, their mothers hovering hawkishly over them, or, alternatively, one of the hollow shells of children who'd been beaten, burned, and maimed within an inch of their lives by their parents or caretakers.

She hoarded sleep when she could get it, in the darkened backs of lecture halls, on the cheap, scratchy couches in the residents' lounge, and in the frigid bunk beds of the call room when she could get there. She hoarded dreamless sleep in particular, since her REM had lately been playing movie-show horrors—an unanesthetized surgery in which the patient was her mother, a gruesome dissection of her own maggoty foot, a hallway full of dead patients she had forgotten to check on or medicate.

She hoarded time like a child's paperclip chain—in the bathroom, in the stairwell between floors, in any crevice where she could pause and not be noticed. Her beepers she did not hoard but fingered intermittently to be reassured of their presence. Were they on? Yes, yes.

She hoarded each breath. In and out. Her chest still moving air into her lungs, her heart still pumping blood in its undulating dance of systole and diastole. She hoarded her legs and their ability to run, her back's ability to hold her body up, her brain which raced amazingly, frenetically along.

She hoarded herself, and the image of a drawn, worried face glimpsed fleetingly in darkened middle-of-the-night windows. And she longed to hold that girl close, even as she slipped slowly from her grasp.

PAS DE DEUX

Danielle Ofri

It was on a desolate winter evening that I escaped from Bellevue. I plunged the last IV of my day into someone's vein and then hopped on an M-15 bus uptown, pressing my subway token into the slot with both anxiety and relief.

I was in the second year of my internal medicine residency training, the middle year, which is marked by what is charitably called a "dip" in motivation. More accurately, it is a pit, a chasm, an abyss, a Stygian marsh. Too far from the newness of internship, too bogged down to see the horizon of future possibilities that senior residents can sense, second-year residents slog through the endless year with their heads down in the muck of monotony. Second year is notorious for depression, doubts, and a generalized dreary outlook on life.

For me, second year was particularly bleak. Having extended medical school to seven years from the usual four in order to complete my

PhD, and then having continued straight through to residency in the same institution, I felt as though I were being buried alive in Bellevue Hospital. The final year of my decade of training seemed eons away, and I was overwhelmed with the drudgery of hospital life. AIDS had saturated our training, and in those days before protease inhibitors and HIV "cocktails," the wards of Bellevue were overflowing with patients my own age dying protracted and miserable deaths. Every day felt the same—legions of feverish, emaciated patients admitted from the emergency room, many with lives as ragged as the Kaposi sarcoma lesions that ulcerated their limbs, mouths, lungs, and intestines. There was a Third World feel to our existence, a soul-numbing tedium of affliction and despair. When the alarm shuddered me out of sleep each morning, I found myself paralyzed in the predawn darkness, trapped in a tangle of grisly dream fragments and a penetrating dread of the upcoming day. I needed to escape.

The M-15 bus chugged through the evening traffic of First Avenue, past the Bellevue Men's Shelter, that crumbling brick behemoth that was the starting point and ending point for so many of my patients. It rumbled past the medical school, where I'd spent innumerable hours in windowless classrooms memorizing details about the pentose phosphate shunt and microtubule organizing centers that had yet to contribute to a single clinical situation in my current life. We passed the United Nations, a gleaming tower that seemed worlds away from Bellevue, except when Tibetan hunger strikers were forcibly brought to our ER.

Wintertime was the worst. Not only was it the midpoint of the middle year, but we would not glimpse sunlight for weeks on end. The cold weather drove the homeless into the hospital, and all of Bellevue seemed a fetid, overcrowded, wretched purgatory to which we were committed until the end of our residency . . . if ever that would arrive.

Sometime during the grim December depths, vague rumblings of a distant childhood desire poked plaintively into my consciousness. As a teenager, I had taken after-school dance classes. I remembered the pleasure of physical movement, the joy of accomplishment, though all that had been fettered shut throughout the straitjacket of college and medical school. The only physical challenges I experienced now involved hauling stretchers to Radiology when there were no transporters available. In the midst of my current dispirited existence, my body seemed to be telling me something. Like a resurrected itch in a difficult spot, something in me ached to reach back to that experience.

Still unsure of even conceptualizing a plan, I'd plunked open the Manhattan yellow pages and perused the long list of dance schools. There were schools of ballet, jazz, modern, ballroom, African, and Latin dance. Some were prestigious professional schools affiliated with major dance companies, some were independent studios, some were solo operations run by individual entrepreneurial dancers. Given the overwhelming selection, I was forced to apply the standard New York City decision-making algorithm: public transportation proximity. The school had to be exactly one subway or bus ride from Bellevue—no transfers or connections.

From my East Side location, the choices quickly boiled down to one, the Martha Graham School of Contemporary Dance. I had vague recollections of melodramatic poses, pelvic contractions, and overwrought eyeshadow, but my time and energy were extremely limited, and I couldn't be picky.

The bus deposited me near a run-down, three-story brick building on East 63rd Street. Zealous ivy blanketed the walls all the way to the roof, though someone had thoughtfully trimmed the leaves around the casement windows. Towering wrought-iron posts enclosed a weedy, overgrown garden. The more eastern edge was bordered by the exit ramp from the Queensboro Bridge, and cars spilled around the corner from Queens with commutational fervor.

Inside the building was a sagging wooden staircase lined with pictures of Martha Graham. There she was in one poster—in a dramatically flowing gown, leg swept frighteningly high overhead in defiance of conventional anatomy, sending cascades of rippled cloth tumbling downward. There she was in another—body crouched into a taut coil, eyes flashing with fiercely blackened outlines, hair amassed in a towering bun, trembling with the rage of Ariadne. Further along was a company photo of dancers flying into the air with the innocent delight of *Appalachian Spring*—skirts billowing from captured air, arms aloft with muscular momentum. The camera had caught all fifteen dancers aloft in midair, and prosaic issues of floors and walls and gravity did not seem of concern.

I tiptoed into the long, narrow studio and parked myself in the far corner, hiding myself as best I could within the curve of the baby grand piano. Thirty students in four long rows stretched and chatted, twisting legs and backs into what struck me as rather medically risky positions. I reached down to touch my toes and something snapped in my back.

Someone evidently glimpsed the teacher in the hallway and everyone scurried into proper first position—dancers ready to perform. The teacher sailed in, her sleek, six-foot-two-inch frame clad in a glistening turquoise unitard. She looked to be in her fifties, with a regal bearing and an effortless elegance of movement. She diligently surveyed the students, examined their posture, adjusted a few stray limbs, then broke into an effervescent grin. "Good ev-en-ing," she declared, with a precise European articulation. "Please be seat-ed." I learned later that this was Armgard, the legendary German instructor of the evening class.

In precise synchrony, without any direction from the teacher, the students extended pointed toes to one side, swept their legs in curved circles, and glided to the ground in an organized, graceful swoop. Startled, I quickly plopped myself onto the floor. The ancient wooden planks were polished smooth from a half century of dancers' bare feet.

I waited patiently for instructions to descend from above; residency had trained me to follow orders well. I was looking forward to being instructed how to dance—this was the Level I class, after all.

No words came, however. With a slight nod from the teacher, the pianist creaked forward on his ancient roller bench and started up on the battered Steinway. Armgard stood silently while the students proceeded uniformly into a set of graceful first position stretches. Precisely eight measures later they simultaneously remodeled their bodies into second position. On they went, without any instruction or cue, executing a complicated set of exercises, shifting to a new position every eight measures. I lurched my eyes toward the teacher, pleading for help, but she was busy counting out the timing. The class moved seamlessly through the sequence, all in tune, all in line. Except for me.

I craned my neck to snatch clues from the students around me. Left arm extended, right leg folded inward. No, now the left leg was folded, right leg straight, torso extended forward. Then back pulled upwards, arms overhead. My limbs flailed like those of a disoriented octopus as I tried to imitate my classmates. The massive wall of mirrors reassured me that I looked as ridiculous as I felt. There was no place to hide.

The first exercise finished, Armgard turned to the pianist. "Could you do something a bit Mozart? A minuet, perhaps?" And the class, once again, launched into a stunningly beautiful set of exercises, without any guidance.

I had been told this was Level I. Where were the instructions? Where was the gentle guidance from the teacher? This was worse than my first day of internship or even the first day of kindergarten. I wanted to shout out, "I am actually a doctor! In real life I am a professional who is accorded responsibility over people's lives."

But my silent entreaties stuttered forlornly onto the worn wooden floor. Everyone else was dancing.

Armgard stopped to correct a student in the second row. "Isn't it remarkable that God gave us two legs instead of one," she said. "Now wouldn't it be helpful if you used *both* of them in the *grand plié?*"

Later on in the class, as things grew more complicated, Armgard began to call out directions. It was hopeless for me, as the music and movement swirled faster than my brain could possibly process. There were far too many limbs to keep track of, and none of mine seemed to be anywhere near the right places at the right time. Armgard was busy repeating her instructions in French, Spanish, and Portuguese as I sank into horrible humiliation. She called out "right" and "left" in Japanese and then Korean, while the pianist spun out seamless variations on Schubert, Bach, Broadway tunes, and the occasional Mick Jagger song that I suspected Armgard didn't recognize.

After class I dashed out of the building, barreling through the crowd of leotard-clad dancers toward the beckoning anonymity of First Avenue so that no one would see my quivering eyes. I don't think I cried even on the first day of kindergarten, but now I was biting my lips to keep back the tears. A doctor, I told myself. You're a full-fledged doctor. With a PhD to boot. My throat trembled nevertheless and threatened to unleash a deluge.

The bridge traffic hurtled across 63rd Street—cars honking, buses careening between lanes, taxis screeching to pick up fares. Bicycle messengers swooped between the cars with dizzying disdain for their own lives, much less anyone else's. A lone traffic cop was inserted into the mess of horns and tires and exhaust fumes, trying to sustain order.

It's just a lousy dance class, I insisted. Probably no one else in that studio would know how to treat diabetic ketoacidosis, right? None of those long-limbed, double-jointed creatures could sink a central line in the jugular vein without dropping a lung, right? But the vision of the class as a single supple organism delicately descending into a unified *plié* trickled over me, cinching my breath with its beauty. Nothing at Bellevue was that beautiful. How could I even think to bring my clomping self, pockets stuffed with ungraceful, unbeautiful Bellevue paraphernalia, into that same space?

I was sure that back in the studio, the teacher was shaking her head in dismay. The other class members were probably snickering in the dressing room. Martha Graham, so elegantly captured in those posters, was probably mourning the decline of her school's artistic standards.

The coarse pavement slapped against my feet as I stomped down First Avenue. I would never, *ever* subject myself to such embarrassment again. The closest I would come to the dance would be as a holder of a ticket stub at Lincoln Center, thank you very much.

The next morning I awoke with a nettled hangover of humiliation. It lumbered along with me as I rounded on my miserable, dying patients. I would *never* return to that building on East 63rd Street.

But then the startling grace of thirty dancers unfurling their left arms skyward, their gaze tipping off the edges of their fingertips, would catch me in the middle of drawing blood and my breath would momentarily halt. Then my reflection in that unforgivingly expansive mirror would pop back at me, my arms and legs straggling like overcooked spaghetti, and I'd peevishly return to my blood draw.

For two days I wrestled with this queer juxtaposition of sensations.

The harder I tried to purge the vestiges of humiliation, the more persistently these longings for beauty nudged forward.

Slowly, oddly, it became clear: I wanted to go back.

Never before had I felt a desire to return to a scene of such mortification, but now I wanted to go back. I wanted that beauty. If I were to survive Bellevue, I *needed* that beauty.

I gathered up my shaky ego, pulled on the leotard that didn't hide a damn thing, and dragged myself back. The second class was still a struggle, but one or two positions felt familiar from the previous class. I recognized the curvature of one arm and managed to get mine there before the movement was entirely over. By the third *plié* I caught up to the music. By the fourth I was there with the rest of the class, my body lowering with the group. In the mirror I caught a peek of the class easing downward and then pulling up, the space above our heads expanding, then contracting. The pianist's fingers softened the notes on the *plié*, then built them up on *relevé*. The choreography and the architecture, the music and the dancers—they interwove to create something that I couldn't describe. Something that gave me a peculiar ache in my chest, an ache that was somehow soothing in its strain, an ache of desire for this delicacy.

I attended class the following week, amazed that I could manage a few of the steps. The long gray days at Bellevue seemed to move a few degrees more quickly. Even though the evening class—ninety-minute lesson, plus commuting each way—added hours to my already long day, it was the only thing that kept my head above the depressing waters of illness and death.

Each day, as soon as I completed the last task on my scut list, I would dash out of Bellevue with a leotard under my scrubs. Exhaustion was my permanent companion during that second year of residency and I would usually fall asleep on the M-15 bus going uptown, but my eyes would open when I'd bring myself into the lush aesthetic of the Graham studio. Sleekly clad in shimmering leotards, hair gracefully swept back, the dancers were the paragon of elegance to me after a full day with my shaggy, sleep-deprived hospital colleagues. The students casually stretched their long limbs in the narrow hallways, chatting in Italian, German, or Korean. The topics of discussion were Juilliard scholarships and Bolshoi performances, not potassium levels or sputum smears. The frenetic dissonance of Bellevue would melt away as the music began, and I would sink gratefully into first position.

I began to attend class regularly, and the movements that had so discombobulated me on that first day now began to grow familiar. As I worked diligently to acquire this new language of movement, the days themselves grew longer, the permanent darkness of winter finally receding. The classes now started in daylight, and the sun would begin its descent while we were dancing. Each time the class sank into a *plié*, an extra beam of fading sunlight succeeded in traversing the room, and then would be shadowed off when the class rose up. The low-angled light cast gentle shadows from "Martha's Garden"—the hodgepodge of shrubs and trees just outside of Studio I. Through windows now opened a crack, tendrils of the wall-climbing vines would snake their way inwards and dangle jauntily near the piano.

Over the course of my second and third years of residency I attended class religiously. It took only a few weeks to become familiar with most of the basic movements, but I soon discovered that there was infinite depth to each one and understood why dancers trained for a lifetime. I also discovered that nature had endowed me with a body that could never do many of the things that Ms. Graham had envisioned. Toes pointing inward, inflexible hip joints, stiff spinal vertebrae constituted my inheritance. Luckily for Martha, though, she was dead and could never witness my perversion of her technique.

I was intrigued by the other students in the class. Half were young dancers attempting to forge a career in performing arts. These were the "trainees" who were officially enrolled in the Martha Graham program. They came from all over the world on student visas and attended class on artistic scholarships. Their superior abilities and professional aspirations were clearly evident.

In many ways, they were not that different from the interns and residents in my medical training program. The fierce—sometimes competitive—determination felt familiar, except that they were striving to master a physical and aesthetic domain instead of a medical one.

The rest of the students exhibited a different type of determination. The dedicated lay folk were teachers, interior designers, nurses, musicians, actors, even a physics professor. They ranged in age and body habitus across a blessedly normal spectrum. They were well aware that nothing short of divine intervention or creative orthopedic surgery would ever turn them into "real" dancers. Yet they were driven by a personal connection to dance for which the word "hobby" would not do justice. Many came every single day after work, even on Saturdays, devoting almost every hour of their free time to this pursuit. Partly, this was because of Armgard. Armgard was uncompromising in her expectations. She knew that every dancer, no matter his or her innate ability, could be pushed to a higher level, and she respected the driving spirit of each one. There was one middle-aged fellow even more awkward than I. He could barely straighten his knees and he was bereft of any sense of musical timing. Yet he came day in and day out, unfazed by the legions of petite, limber dancers around him. Armgard encouraged him as much as she did the students who were bound for the professional world. In Armgard's class, we all felt like we were dancing.

Almost every dancer was outfitted with a unitard that Armgard sewed in her apartment—the same ones she sewed for the members of the actual Martha Graham Dance Company. I remember the surge of pride I felt when I finally got an Armgard unitard. I chose turquoise, the same color that Armgard had worn on my very first day. I could be a dancer too.

No matter how drained or reluctant I felt on any given night, Armgard's class always left my body rippling with alertness, and that awareness pulled me to the studio every day after my hospital work was done, no matter how exhausted I was. My biggest regret was missing class when I was on call overnight. During those late nights I would sometimes find myself alone in one of the long, empty halls of Bellevue. The temptation of open space would be too much. I would peek at each end to ensure that no one was coming and then let loose in my private studio. *Chassé* turns and triplets, high leaps and barrel turns, all the exuberant moves my small apartment could not accommodate. My stethoscope still has the gash it received when it catapulted out of my white coat during one of the more energetic spins. One janitor experienced an angina episode when his mop and my *glissade* collided.

One day, after a long night in the ICU, I rushed straight from Bellevue to dance class rather than going home to sleep. I had spent the bulk of my last thirty hours with Nilsa, a young woman dying of HIV. Up until that night she had been on the regular ward in the end stages of her disease. She no longer had any awareness of herself and her family had signed a Do Not Resuscitate order. For reasons that were unknown to me, the DNR order had been rescinded earlier that day. Nilsa was shipped off to the ICU so that "everything could be done."

Nilsa's body was ravaged by bacterial, viral, and fungal infections. The body cavities that weren't drowning in their own fluids were hemorrhaging blood. Her temperature never dipped below 103°. The breathing machine provided oxygen in exchange for her tuberculosis-laden breaths. I was frustrated that some other doctor had somehow given the family a false sense of hope and encouraged them to rescind the DNR. With my limited Spanish I tried to explain to the family the futility of the situation, but the point rapidly became moot; Nilsa's body slowly gave out. I injected sedatives when she convulsed, her water-logged lungs laboring to absorb more oxygen. The nurse and I arranged icepacks around her burning skin, but they melted rapidly. Her death was slow and brutal. Her mother, two brothers, and aunt sat with her, weeping into their protective respiratory masks.

I limped out of the hospital after signing Nilsa's death certificate. There were so many infections that I couldn't decide which one to write for "immediate cause of death." My sleep-starved body longed for bed, but my aching soul dragged my protesting limbs to East 63rd Street.

We were doing the *plié-relevé* series, a set of exercises that I have always found particularly beautiful. There is one point, in fifth position, in which the drama builds until the climax occurs with just one simple motion: a ninety-degree twist of the body while lifting into a *relevé*, one arm scooping an arc into the sky. In one brief but compelling moment, the whole class rises into the air as a single being, sweeping its focus from the one corner of the room to the other. Physically subtle, yet emotionally dramatic, almost more so for the understatement of the movement.

On that night, I struggled to keep my weary muscles in line. The music was surging, and the intensity of the dance was rising. It culminated in this modest, but so powerful, shift of the body. Something peaked in me. The music and the movement were suddenly too hauntingly beautiful to tolerate. Too painfully gorgeous to share space in my soul with Nilsa's death. Putrid secretions, purulent sores, bloated limbs, vomited blood: these were the cadences of Nilsa's final hours. How could the beauty enveloping me now exist in the same universe with such agony? I could not contain them both. They ruptured inside as I melted onto the bare wooden floor, my hacking sobs a dissonant counterpoint to the music.

Medical training is, in many ways, like a disease. Over the course of medical history, treatments have been devised to rescue patients from other fatal diseases: patients with hemophilia are kept alive with repeated infusions of a crucial clotting factor into their veins. Patients with sickle cell disease require red cell transfusions to stay alive. Patients with end-stage renal disease are kept alive with dialysis.

There are numerous pathologies in the disease of medical training—sleep deprivation, overburdened interns, error-prone systems, social isolation, debasing hierarchy. Many of these pathologies have begun to be addressed, but I discovered that there was another that had not (yet) been the subject of a blue-ribbon commission or a well-publicized lawsuit—the absence of beauty. Perhaps in the grand scheme of the scourges of residency, this seems like only a minor misery. But for me, it took a palpable toll, one that I wasn't even aware of until the "treatment" started helping me. I look back now and realize that it was the continual infusion of the aesthetics of dance that helped keep me alive through those draining years. After each daily dose of agony and suffering, I needed not only to witness beauty but to participate in beauty. I was well aware that I couldn't possibly approach the feats of the advanced dancers, but that turned out not to matter at all. It was enough just to be a bit player in that world, to be a minuscule stitch in that weave of beauty.

In figuring out what type of doctor I wanted to be, I had many earnest advisers in the medical field. They advised me about fellowships, practice settings, and academics. They tried to help me figure out whether I might be better suited to nephrology versus oncology, or academic medicine versus private practice, but to me these didn't feel like the pressing questions. I'd happily have rolled a pair of dice, and I knew that I could make myself comfortable in any field.

It was the addition of dance to my medical training, it seemed, that informed my career path more than all of that well-meaning but ultimately inadequate advice. Somehow, I would have to shape my medical life so that it could encompass the arts and the humanities. This was a radical departure not only from my colleagues but also from my academic career thus far. I'd been on the straight and narrow scientific path ever since I'd wanted to be a veterinarian in elementary school. I could never have imagined that the squishy arts might occupy a front row seat next to the hard sciences. But then again, I didn't plan this path; it just unfurled itself this way.

Dance followed my medical career for many years, and the Martha Graham School was an integral part of my life. After I had children, the logistics of evening classes became impossible. But during some travels after residency finished, I'd started jotting down my medical experiences. This grew into a stronger focus as I began to take writing classes. Eventually I gathered my writings into two books. Later, I helped start the *Bellevue Literary Review*, and found myself knee-deep in poetry, short stories, and essays between my clinic sessions. I started handing out poems to unsuspecting interns, elevator reading to break the monotony of medicine.

When my daughter started violin lessons, I matter-of-factly asked the teacher how best to encourage practicing. She shrugged and replied that it often helped for kids to see their parents play music. A week later, I purchased a student cello and started lessons. What began as a parental exercise in pedagogy quickly became a passion, and I found myself studying music more intensively than I'd ever studied for my medical boards.

Looking back at the unplanned hodgepodge of dance, literature, and music in my life, I realize that I can't be a doctor without this creative aspect, despite remaining forever an amateur in each field. The middle of my residency was as close as I'd ever come to drowning in the morass of medicine. To be whole, I somehow need both—the two serpents entwined in the medical caduceus symbol, partners in the *pas de deux*.

There are times, as I slog through this messy business of illness and dying, when I fantasize about the beautiful world of dance, where the only concerns are the clean architectural lines of the body and the aesthetic qualities of the movement. I know that a professional artistic career is far more arduous than I could possibly contemplate, but from the medical trenches it shimmers seductively.

It seems to me no accident that the ritual healings of many societies have involved dance. There is a physical intimacy of healing that has been recognized for thousands of years. This has been diminished in modern times due to the myriad diagnostic tools of modern medicine, but it doggedly persists. The physical exam might be described as its own *pas de deux* between doctor and patient; medical visits that lack a physical exam often leave patients feeling as though something is missing. I am no Luddite, and I would certainly feel bereft without MRIs and computerized medical databases, but I am repeatedly impressed by the power of connection that occurs via touch. The laying on of hands represents the unalloyed physicality of medicine that is a resonant partner with dance.

Sometimes, in the middle of a busy day, when my frustration is rising and the sense of being overwhelmed threatens to choke me, I'll suddenly notice that my feet have crept into fifth position. My body will unconsciously realign itself, shifting my upper body to balance against my lower, unfurling a breath that sheds some of the accumulated angst. I'll often feel compelled to reach over and touch my patient on the arm, and then I'll feel my mind begin to unsnarl. I can sense it beginning to clear, just enough to focus on what the patient is saying, just enough to connect to the person who is sharing this space and this moment with me. For we are nothing if not partners in an intimate dance.

FIRST IN MY CLASS

Chris Stookey

I was an average resident. My national board scores were near the middle percentile; my technical skills were neither stellar nor inadequate; if anything, I suppose my bedside manner was my forte. However, there was one area in which I stood out. I had the distinction of being the first member of my residency class to be successfully sued for medical malpractice. In fact, I may have been one of the youngest individuals ever named to the NPDB, the National Practitioner Data Bank. The NPDB is a list of all the health care providers in the United States who have been successfully sued for malpractice—every physician, nurse, midwife, chiropractor, herbalist, osteopath, physical therapist, and acupuncturist who's ever lost or settled a malpractice case for a dollar amount equal to or exceeding one cent. The list may be obtained by anyone who wants it. There's a convenient Internet Web site; all you have to do is run a search on the name of the practitioner you're interested in. You'll forgive me if I don't provide the relevant Web address—if you want a look at the list, I'll leave you to your own research.

My own case involved a patient I saw during the second month of my residency. At the time, I hadn't known you could sue a resident for malpractice. I figured, as residents, we were protected under the wings of the attending physicians who supervised our work. I was wrong about that.

The first news of the lawsuit came in the form of a letter delivered to my mailbox in the residents' lounge. I was doing my rotation in surgery, putting in sixteen hours a day plus every third night on call in the emergency room. I wandered into the lounge that afternoon after having spent the morning holding retractors in the OR on a colon case. Immediately upon seeing the distinctly marked envelope in my box, I had a bad feeling. The return address read *LAW OFFICES: QUENTIN, CARGILL, KETTLE, & AMES.* The letter was addressed using my full name, sent in care of the medical center hospital. Most conspicuous of all were the words written just to the left of my name, three words written in bold, underlined, capital letters:

PERSONAL AND CONFIDENTIAL

I glanced around the room. I was alone. Tearing open the envelope, I unfolded the letter and read:

Dear Dr. Stookey:

This firm has been appointed to defend you and all other entities in the matter Nguyen v. The University of XXX. You were a treating physician in this case which involves alleged medical malpractice.

If you have not already done so, I would appreciate your creating a file separate from any medical records concerning this claimant. Please do not discuss this case with anyone other than myself or members of my firm. As long as you limit your communications this way, it is likely you will be protected under attorney/client privilege. If you receive a subpoena relating to the case, notify me immediately. Finally, please do not undertake any independent investigation regarding this action, either as to the facts which gave rise to it or as to the medical issues.

I will need to be in contact with you throughout the duration of this litigation. It is important that I meet with you at your earliest possible convenience for an initial interview. Please contact my secretary who will set up a meeting at a time and location suitable to your schedule.

Very truly yours,
Leslie R. Mazzella
Attorney at Law

My first reaction was disbelief. In fact, I imagined the letter had to be a malicious prank perpetrated by one of my fellow interns. Just the day before, another intern had handed me a phone, saying it was the coroner, who wanted to talk to me about one of my "former" patients (the call was actually from a nurse who wanted a clarification on an insulin order). But, reading through the letter a second time, I could see there was a disquieting ring of truth to it all, from the formal letterhead to the scratchy blue-ink signature.

Alleged medical malpractice. Christ, I was being sued.

I shoved the letter in my pocket. In five minutes I was scheduled to be in surgery clinic, where I had a full afternoon's booking of patients to see. However, rather than head to the clinic, I went to the Quad, the grassy area between the two wings of the medical center. I needed to get outside for a minute and breathe some fresh air.

Sitting on the grass, I read through the letter again. I noted there were no details concerning the nature of the case, nothing about what

I was being sued for. The only thing I'd been given was a name: *Nguyen*. I tried to remember. Nguyen. The name rang no bells, ominous or otherwise. I tried to recall a patient I'd seen who'd had a bad outcome, a case that had taken a disastrous turn. Of course, there'd been patients with the usual complications, but there was no case that stood out, no particular patient who'd prompted me to think: "God, this is going to end up in a lawsuit." Nguyen. The letter didn't even indicate if Nguyen was a man or a woman.

My pager went off. It was the surgery clinic wondering where I was. I stuffed the letter in my pocket and headed for the outpatient building.

The clinic that afternoon seemed interminable. I couldn't stop thinking about the letter. I moved in a daze, walking once into the wrong room and confusing a pre-op physical for a post-op wound check. I kept trying to remember. Nguyen. Nguyen. Between a wound dressing change and a suture removal on a child, I slipped into the bathroom and reread the letter yet again. *You were a treating physician* . . . What possibly could have happened? Had I missed a critical diagnosis, mistaken an appendicitis for a stomach flu, diagnosed rib pain in a patient having a heart attack?

The clinic finished up at 6 p.m. I still had to make evening rounds with the surgery inpatient team before going home. Stepping from the elevator onto the surgical floor of the main hospital, I should have started immediately into my pre-rounding work. Instead, I went over to one of the computer terminals and typed in a patient name search. *N-g-u-y-e-n*. I took a deep breath and pressed ENTER.

There were twenty-six people with the name Nguyen in the hospital data bank. Aaron Nguyen, Alice Nguyen, Bernard Nguyen . . . One of those Nguyens was my Nguyen. One of those Nguyens was suing me for malpractice. I read through all twenty-six names, down to Yvonne Nguyen. None of the names struck a chord.

My pager went off again. The surgical team was waiting for me. I abandoned my Nguyen search and headed off to rounds.

I got home to my apartment at ten o'clock that night. Sitting down at the table in my kitchen, I read through the Mazzella letter once again (how many times would I read that letter?). I noted now the many admonitions: don't discuss the case with anyone, don't undertake an independent investigation of the medical "issues" (why had the plural been used here?), don't respond to any subpoena.

I had a hard time getting to sleep that night. My mind swam through a heaving sea of Nguyen scenarios gone bad: a fracture missed on X-ray, an overlooked lab result, an infected wound, a preventable blood clot. Nguyen had died. Or, worse, Nguyen had become permanently disabled. I imagined a middle-aged, unisex Nguyen existing in a nursing home on a ventilator, paralyzed, tethered to a tangle of tubes invading every orifice.

The numbers on the digital clock next to my bed progressed inexorably forward: 1:30, 2:00, 2:30. Morning rounds began in just four hours. I had to get some sleep. But my mind would not let go of the parade of horrors: missed breast lump, bleeding from the colon attributed to "just hemorrhoids." Was Nguyen young or old? God, what if Nguyen was a child?

Sometime after three o'clock I dozed off—only to be awoken by the alarm blaring in my ear at five fifteen.

After rounds and duties on the surgical floor that next morning, I snuck away and phoned Leslie Mazzella. I didn't want to make the call on the ward where the nurses and doctors could hear me. I still hadn't spoken to anyone about the case. After all, Mazzella's letter had warned, *Please do not discuss this case with anyone.* So, I went downstairs to the pay phones in the hospital lobby.

My heart pounded as I dialed the number. Although I was burning to know more about the case, I was also sick to my stomach in anticipation of learning the precise charges against me. A young woman answered the phone: "Quentin & Cargill."

"Yes, I'm Chris Stookey. May I speak to Ms. Maz—"

"Oh, yes, Dr. Stookey."

"Christ," I thought, "she knows who I am." I'd imagined Quentin & Cargill as some busy law firm located in a high-rise glass tower downtown. Yet the secretary had immediately recognized my name. It was as though she'd been sitting at her desk waiting for my call.

"I, uh, received a letter."

"Yes, Ms. Mazzella would like to set up an initial interview regarding the Nguyen case." She said it so nonchalantly—*the Nguyen case.* I made note of the phrase, "initial interview" (Mazzella's letter had used the same phrase): it carried the implication of the first in a series. "Is there a day that would be convenient for you?"

"Yes, well—may I speak to Ms. Mazzella?"

"She's in a deposition today. She's free tomorrow, however—she could meet you at the hospital."

My anxiety ratcheted up another notch. Tomorrow. So soon? They weren't wasting any time. "Well, I suppose . . . at lunchtime."

"All right. Twelve o'clock at the hospital? Where's a good place to meet?"

"Well—how about . . . the library?" I said. "We could use one of the study rooms. They're pretty private."

"Perfect. I'll let Ms. Mazzella know. She'll meet you tomorrow at twelve at the entrance to the hospital library."

I was about to hang up, but I had to ask. "Say—"

"Yes?"

"Could you—?"

"Yes?"

"The Nguyen case. What's it about, anyway?"

"Oh, Ms. Mazzella will fill you in on everything tomorrow."

"But, I mean . . . What . . . Did someone die?"

"It's really not my place to discuss the details, Dr. Stookey. I'm sure you understand."

"Yes. Yes, of course."

"Ms. Mazzella will fill you in on everything tomorrow."

I slept poorly again that night, once again falling asleep after 3 a.m. When I awoke in the morning, I had a sore throat and felt achy all over. I have a tendency to get physically ill during times of emotional stress. I took my temperature: 100.1. No doubt about it, I was coming down with something.

On morning rounds, the attending physician mentioned I looked a little "peaked." I felt nauseated, and my voice was becoming hoarse. I was assigned to light duty: third assist on a gallbladder case. The principal surgeon was a second-year resident, and it was only his second cholecystectomy. The operation started at nine, and the going was slow. Standing there holding retractors and suctioning, I kept looking at the clock. By eleven fifteen, we still hadn't begun to close the case. The gallbladder was out, but the second year wanted to take a minute to "look around at the anatomy."

Due to my fever, I found myself sweating profusely during the operation. The scrub nurse kept wiping my forehead. "Are you all right?" she asked several times. Finally, at 11:45 a.m., we finished the case. I left the operating suite and bolted for the showers.

I arrived at the library at precisely twelve o'clock. My hair was wet from the shower, and beads of water dripped down the side of my face. I'd changed into a fresh pair of green scrubs. A minute later, a woman—fortyish, immaculate in a blue suit, carrying a leather briefcase—walked hurriedly up to the entrance. I immediately knew it was Mazzella; she had a lawyer's face and a lawyer's demeanor: intelligent, genteel, predatory. I, too, must have had the anticipated appearance. The moment she saw me, she blurted out: "Dr. Stookey!" She reached out her hand. "Leslie Mazzella."

"Hi," I croaked. "Chris Stookey."

"Touch of laryngitis, Chris?"

"Oh . . . I think I'm getting a cold."

"You should see a doctor. Plenty of those around here!"

I forced a chuckle.

"So," Mazzella said, "is there a place to sit down?"

We went inside the library and found an empty cubicle. Sitting down at the table, Mazzella opened her briefcase and took out a six-inch-thick, bound folder.

"Now," she said opening the folder, "just how much do you recall about Jill Nguyen, a patient you saw six months ago, on August 12?"

My world tilted a little. *Jill* Nguyen. So—Nguyen was a woman. I still didn't remember the name. I brushed back my wet hair. "Nothing," I said. "I don't remember her."

"Good," Mazzella said. "*Tabula rasa*, that's the way I like it." She began flipping through the pages of her folder. "You only saw her the one time. She was admitted to the obstetrical floor, eight months pregnant."

My world tilted again, and my stomach tightened. *Pregnant?* This was completely unexpected, something I hadn't considered in even my darkest Nguyen scenarios. *Pregnant?*

Mazzella continued. "Her prenatal care was sporadic. She missed two routine prenatal appointments. She was admitted to the OB floor on August 12 for labor contractions, placed on the usual monitors.

The fetal heart tracing suggested some problems. Any of this ring a bell?"

"No," I said. "Not at all."

"A decision was made to send Mrs. Nguyen for a biophysical profile. As I'm sure you know, that's an ultrasound test to measure parameters of fetal well-being: heart rate, breathing rate, limb movements. The plan was to move to an early Cesarean section if the profile was poor. Apparently, your involvement was pretty brief. There's not much documentation, just something in the nurse's notes." Mazzella flipped to a tagged page in her folder. "Something about Mrs. Nguyen having a red eye. Here it is." Mazzella folded back the page and slid the folder across the table.

Halfway down the tagged page was a brief entry in the nurse's notes, highlighted in yellow: *12:10. Dr. Stookey at bedside to examine red left eye.*

It was then the light switched on inside my head. Of course, *Mrs. Nguyen.* I remembered her now. Suddenly, there she was, plain as day: a young, petite, Asian woman on the OB deck, sweat on her forehead, a pained facial grimace during a labor contraction. Yes, Mrs. Nguyen, the pregnant woman with the red eye. It was my second month as an intern, and I was doing my obstetrical rotation, spending the month on the OB floor delivering babies. Mrs. Nguyen had not been one of my patients—she belonged to another intern. But I'd walked by her room just as she was about to leave for the biophysical profile Mazzella had mentioned. Mrs. Nguyen had called out as I walked by: "There's a doctor. Can he look at it?"

The OB nurse called me into the room and explained Mrs. Nguyen was concerned about a painless red area that had developed in her left eye. I looked at the eye. The outer, lower quadrant of the white part of the eye was red. The diagnosis was easy. Mrs. Nguyen had a subconjunctival hematoma. A small blood vessel on the surface of the eye had burst, resulting in some bleeding into the lower surface of the eye. It was a common condition and entirely benign. Most likely, the straining Mrs. Nguyen was doing during her labor had caused the ruptured blood vessel. I reassured her about the condition, telling her it was nothing serious. The blood would gradually fade away, and the eye would be back to its normal white color in a few days. The nurse then mentioned the concern regarding Mrs. Nguyen's labor and said Mrs. Nguyen was about to leave for the profile test. I said, by all means, go for the test—nothing needed to be done about the eye. And that was it. That was the full extent of my interaction with Jill Nguyen.

I explained all this to Mazzella, who rubbed her chin. "Hmm . . . ," she said. She turned to the next page in her folder. "Well . . . do you happen to recall looking at this while you were in the room?"

Mazzella slid her folder across the table again and pointed to a strip of paper. It was a fetal heartbeat tracing. The tracing was highly abnormal. Rather than the regular, spiked heartbeats you expect on a normal tracing, this tracing showed an undulating, sinusoidal pattern. Even a medical student could have instantly recognized this was the heart tracing of a baby in extreme distress. That tracing was what doctors call a "terminal rhythm." It was the tracing of a baby about to die. A baby with that heart tracing needed to be delivered by Cesarean section. Immediately.

"Did you see the tracing?" Mazzella asked again.

"N-no," I said. "I just looked at the eye."

"All right," Mazzella said. "That will be our defense, then."

"Defense?"

"Yes. This was the tracing on the monitor when you were in the room. See the time mark?"

I looked at the time mark on the rhythm strip: 12:10. Precisely the time the nurse's note documented I was in the room. I felt my stomach sink. "But I never looked at the monitor," I said.

"Yes," Mazzella said. "As I say, that will be our defense."

A drop of moisture trickled down my forehead. "W-what happened?" I asked.

Mazzella flipped forward a couple pages in her folder. "Well, when Mrs. Nguyen arrived at the ultrasound suite for the biophysical profile . . . there was no heartbeat. Sometime between the labor room and the ultrasound suite, the baby died."

I stared down at the undulating, sinusoidal heartbeat tracing. The nausea I'd felt throughout the day got suddenly worse, and the moisture was now running down both sides of my forehead. I requested a five-minute time-out and headed for the restroom. I vomited into the sink before I could even reach the toilets.

The rest of the meeting with Mazzella lasted half an hour. Mazzella filled me in on the additional details of the suit. Mrs. Nguyen was suing because she felt a Cesarean section should have been performed immediately. At the point when the biophysical profile was ordered, the baby was already in extreme distress. Only an immediate C-section could have saved the baby's life.

Several other doctors were involved in the suit: the other intern taking care of Nguyen, the resident supervising the interns, the attending physician in charge of obstetrical floor that day. However, as Mazzella made clear, *I* was a key element in the plaintiff's complaint. I was the last person to see Mrs. Nguyen before her baby died. I had been in the room when the fetal heart tracing had gone from "concerning" to "terminal." I had done nothing about it.

They say there are two types of physicians when it comes to the reality of malpractice lawsuits in today's world. Some physicians hardly blink an eye at being named in a suit. It's part of doing business, they say. The average physician gets pulled into a malpractice case once every seven years. Medicine is not an exact science; some patients have bad outcomes. Things go wrong. Lawsuits happen. It's unavoidable. Why worry about it? Just accept what's inevitable and move on.

The second type of physician finds it difficult to be so casual about being sued. At the very least, a lawsuit is a painful, time-consuming nuisance: there are meetings with lawyers, depositions, chart reviews, phone calls, and perhaps even a jury trial. On top of this, being sued for "bad practice" is inevitably a blow to one's self-esteem, a time of embarrassment, humiliation, and self-questioning. Have I made an error so egregious I deserve to be sued over it? Am I *that* incompetent? Do I even belong in this profession?

When I got home that night after the Mazzella meeting, I went straight to bed. My cold was worse: my fever was higher; my throat was on fire; I had stomach cramps. Plus, I was exhausted. I'd gotten less than five hours of sleep over the last two nights.

Yet I still couldn't get to sleep. I couldn't stop thinking about Mrs. Nguyen's baby.

I suppose I might have been a little relieved by what I'd learned from Leslie Mazzella that day. My involvement in the case had been minimal. I'd been asked to look at Mrs. Nguyen's eye. I'd done that. I'd made the proper diagnosis: subconjunctival hematoma. I'd made the proper recommendation: do nothing.

My reaction, however, was not one of relief. My reaction was one of unmitigated remorse. That heart tracing—I *should* have looked at it. Just a brief glance, that's all it would have taken. We were taught to look at the fetal monitor every time we entered the room of a patient in labor. Had I looked, I would have immediately recognized the baby was in deep trouble. I would have notified the senior resident. An emergency Cesarean section would have been performed. The baby might well have been saved.

Over the next several days, my cold got worse, and I had to call in sick. Moreover, my insomnia continued, unabated. Some nights it seemed I didn't get any sleep at all. I just couldn't stop thinking about that baby. I just couldn't stop asking myself: why hadn't I looked at that tracing?

About ten weeks after the meeting in the library, I got a second letter from Leslie Mazzella. Once again, the letter came to my mailbox in the residents' lounge, and once again, the envelope was marked **PER-SONAL AND CONFIDENTIAL**. It was the first I'd heard from Mazzella since our one and only meeting. I took the letter outside to the Quad and sat down on the grass.

> *Dear Dr. Stookey:*
>
> *This letter is to inform you the above referenced matter has been concluded. While the co-defendants continue to believe grounds supporting the accusation of medical malpractice are lacking, the university has decided to settle the case. The university, acting in consultation with this law firm, believes such an out of court settlement is in the best interests of all parties involved.*
>
> *I wish to thank you for your assistance in this matter. I also wish to personally extend my best wishes to you and your future medical career.*
>
> *Sincerely,*
> *Leslie R. Mazzella*
> *Attorney at Law*

It's been nearly two decades now since the Nguyen case. I've stayed with being a doctor, although Mrs. Nguyen and her baby did cause me to question my future as a physician. If I could make a mistake as basic as not looking at a heart tracing, what other mistakes—worse mistakes—would I make over my career?

I still think about them, Mrs. Nguyen and her baby, to this day. That undulating heart tracing still pops into my head from time to time, often at seemingly random moments: while I'm standing in line to get a cup of coffee, listening to music, jogging the fire trails with my dogs. The memory also comes at more predictable times: for example, when I step into an exam room with a pregnant patient.

As to the National Practitioner Data Bank, I have never checked to see if my name got placed on the list after Mazzella settled the case. I've never logged on to the Web site and run a search on my name. The thought of seeing my name pop up—well, what's the point? It wouldn't change anything. Mrs. Nguyen's baby would still have died, and I still would have been the last doctor to examine Mrs. Nguyen while her baby was alive.

If Mrs. Nguyen's baby had lived, she'd be in her late teens now. I say "she" because I learned the baby was a girl (a prenatal ultrasound had determined the sex). Sometimes I wonder what she would have made out of life. Where would she be living? What would she look like? Would she be college bound? Starting a family of her own?

If only I had looked at that tracing.

THE PATIENT NARRATIVE

Perri Klass

Part of my job is to walk into a room and introduce myself to a stranger, and start asking questions. And when I step across that threshold—into another room to meet another stranger and hear another story—I feel myself stepping into my professional identity. Perhaps if I were a surgeon, I would have a more dramatic defining moment: to scrub and glove and gown and walk into the operating room. Perhaps if I were an obstetrician, it would be the rituals of awaiting and then delivering a new life which would remind me: this is who you are, this is what you do. But I do primary care, and I have no special chamber, no glittering instruments, no recurring moments at the bloody boundaries of life. What I have is that everyday threshold, across which you step to enter the zone of the patient and the patient's story.

In the fall, I work with a group (or a couple of groups) of first-year medical students, and I take those steps with them into patients' rooms. Like many medical schools, mine makes an attempt to loop you all the way round, in that very first year, when you are still up to your neck (or any other body part, as the case may be, depending on the curriculum) in gross anatomy. Our attempt is "the patient narrative," part of a larger course on the patient, the physician, and society. And in the patient narrative meetings, as I take a small group in to talk to a patient, the students are supposed to get a sense of what is waiting for them on the other side of gross anatomy and pathophysiology.

I have a son in medical school, in a different institution. I asked him, as he was beginning his second year of medical school, what his classmates say when they come back from their own "clinical exposures," and he told me that people come back and say, "Oh, my God, I can't believe what I saw today." And as soon as he said that, I began to worry about whether I would be able to provide that oh-my-God moment for my own students, and also to hope that my son's clinical preceptor would get it right and serve him up something suitably overwhelming. I wanted him to be floored by the experience of talking to a patient. I wanted it to be unexpected and world-changing in a way that would let him know that he had made the right career choice, but would leave him with renewed respect for all there was to learn. And then I thought about that conversation and that responsibility as I took a group of first-year medical students to meet a patient for the first time.

It's a somewhat calculated attempt to stir them and move them and rock their worlds, and to be honest, like the good students they are, they are generally aware of the goal and prepared to be stirred and moved and rocked. That doesn't make the experience of interviewing a patient any less real, I suppose. In fact, maybe the surprise for me of participating in this course is that *nothing* makes the experience of

interviewing a patient any less real. Here we are, interviewing someone as a group of four students and an attending, with the patient fully
aware that these are students learning to interview—aware, in other
words, that this is an interview about interviewing, not about actually
making medical care decisions. The conventions of the doctor-patient
encounter do not quite seem to apply; we are a study group asking
questions with no clinical intentions, as opposed to a single designated
clinician—even a clinician-in-training—asking questions with a view
toward decision making and therapeutics. And yet, to be in a room
with a stranger, to be asking these questions, to be invited to ask these
questions, to hear the responses and try to piece the story together,
still feels real, and still seems to give some new and different and even
astonishing reality to the experience of being a medical student, and
a beginner.

In the past, the medical students assigned to me have complained
that I tend to take them to see too many pediatric patients, to interview too many parents, occasionally to struggle with adolescents, who
can be somewhat frustrating to interview. So I make good resolutions
about venturing into the adult ward or the hemodialysis unit or the
surgical clinic, but I also want anyone who studies with me to understand the special rhythms of the pediatric interview. And so, with this
particular group of students on their first day, I found myself introduc-
ing them to a father, on the inpatient pediatric ward.

We stood somewhat awkwardly in a semicircle, the four first-year
students and me. We faced "the father," who had agreed to be interviewed by this group. Before we went in to meet him, I had told the students one sentence about his daughter's illness; she was in the hospital
being worked up for osteogenesis imperfecta. None of them had heard
of it, so I took refuge in the conventional cliché: it's the brittle bone
disease, I said. I didn't try to explain the pathophysiology (I like the
way that sentence suggests that of course, I *could* have explained the

pathophysiology, casually off the cuff, if I had been so inclined), and I didn't tell them anything more about this particular child's story.

I find that even as I describe this scene, I reach for the medical convention to describe the child, as if I were presenting the case: almost-two-year-old female with rule/out osteogenesis imperfecta, is what it would say on the residents' sign-out sheet (well, actually, "23mo F r/o OI"). But of course, that wasn't how the father introduced his daughter—or himself. He was a relatively young man, staying in the hospital with his daughter, who had sustained seven broken bones over the course of her short life. She was confined to her stroller, with her leg, in its cast, carefully positioned and elevated. Before we interviewed him, we admired the little girl, who looked at us carefully out of her serious dark eyes, and finally, when her father talked to her, allowed us a guarded smile.

What he wanted to tell us about was what it is like to be a parent whose child is in the process of receiving a serious diagnosis. A parent who has suddenly learned a great deal about a disease he had never even heard of before, so that two Latin words which would have meant nothing to him a couple of weeks ago are now written in fire—or perhaps in blood—across his horizon.

The students asked questions. One of them asked about family history, and he told her proudly about his grandfather back home on the Indian subcontinent, who was over a hundred years old, and "still walks to the mosque." No one else with bone problems. No one else with any problems at all, he said.

He told them about the bumpy road to this diagnosis—he had brought the baby to another hospital, to the emergency room, when she had her first fracture, and they had told him nothing was wrong, they hadn't done an X-ray, and then he and his wife had been so sure that something was wrong, but they had had to go back and protest and insist.

The students asked, somewhat hesitantly, about what the diagnosis would mean for the little girl, if it were confirmed, and he told them that he had been told there was a possibility that her bones might get a little stronger as she got older. But it was clear that he knew that it was a bad disease to live with, and that a small child who has already fractured seven bones in normal everyday childhood activities is probably going to lead a restricted life. Had someone explicitly told him that she might need a wheelchair, that she might need more operations? He didn't say, and certainly I didn't ask, but the emotion in his voice made it clear that he understood that this was a serious illness, that it would change the course of his daughter's life, that nothing would ever be quite the same. And the students got that, and I could see them thinking about it.

He told them that he had a new baby—only a week old, home with his wife, because the hospital ward is not a safe place for babies, since so many children have infectious diseases. And that now the doctors were worrying that the baby should also be checked for osteogenesis imperfecta—this thing, this entity he had never heard of, which was now overshadowing all family joy.

He told them a little about his job history in New York, a job in business, a stint driving a cab, a stint in school.

He told them a little bit about staying in the hospital to keep his daughter company, to wheel her up and down the corridors in her stroller, to make sure that her favorite cartoons were playing—while we talked to him, the baby was watching Dora the Explorer. I hoped the students were getting a little sense of what it is like to live this shadow hospital life; I hoped they were getting a sense of the texture of parental affection; I hoped they were a little bit tantalized by the medical and biochemical and genetic story of a rare disease. But I could also see something else, very clearly, and there is no possible way to put it but this: they were seeing this father as a tragic figure.

They were in a room with someone who was going through something terrible, and even as he asked them to pray for him and pray for his family, and even as they nodded, they also knew it: they have chosen a career which brings them into the room with what is truly important in people's lives, and sometimes what is truly important is difficult and sad and even tragic.

So, after the interview, we went back to a seminar room and sat around a table. We talked about the child's prognosis, and we talked about the father's sadness, and we talked about what was happening to his family. And I found myself saying to them, Look at all the narratives going on in this room, look at all the stories to be told.

There's a genetic story, about a disease which is usually inherited as an autosomal dominant condition, though there is also a recessive form (needless to say, I have since looked all this up and verified my facts), and to meet this father's needs, we would need to understand the process of sorting out the different types of osteogenesis imperfecta, with their different clinical patterns.

There's a biological story of bone development, in which defects in Type I collagen prevent the formation of normal strong bones, and we need to remember that the best hope for therapies which might improve a child's life lies in better understanding of this biology.

There's a child development story about trying to explore the world when rolling over can break your bones, and whenever we think about chronic illness in children, we have to think about how it integrates into development.

There's a family story here, and we always have to think about how illnesses happen to whole families.

There's an immigration story here, a father who came to the United States a decade ago, and worked a variety of jobs, and went home and married and brought his wife back to New York to start a family, and we should think about the life trajectories of our patients and pause, perhaps, to marvel at our own hospital as an international crossroad, and a stop in so many long and complicated journeys.

There's a day-by-day story of a parent living in the hospital, separated from his wife and his newborn baby, tending a little girl tied into a stroller, and we should recognize the role he's playing in her health and her mental health; his world may be tottering, but her world is intact because he's there.

There's probably even a religious story, since the father clearly identifies his faith as the only thing that keeps him going, since he asked you over and over again to pray for his family, and we should never forget to think about where patients get their strength.

And what I was trying to say, I think, was something like this: Look at all these different narratives crossing and weaving together in this encounter—genetics, biochemistry, family, health care system, politics, religion, economics, immigration—and appreciate and acknowledge that you have undertaken to do your job in situations with many different coordinates to be mapped, with narratives that cannot and should not be simplified.

And here they were, the students, at the beginning of medical training. They didn't know the genetics or the biochemistry (neither did I, really, off the top of my head, though I could fake it). They didn't know that osteogenesis imperfecta comes up all the time in pediatrics because it has to be considered in many cases where child abuse is suspected— a more common cause of multiple fractures in a very small child. So there may be a story here of what the medical system put these parents through before anyone realized what was really going on.

And why say all this to students, right at the beginning, before they know what osteogenesis imperfecta is, before they've ever thought about working up a child for possible child abuse, before they've learned any of the information which will one day maybe let them be helpful to a parent in distress? I think we do it almost as an article of faith: it's a way of giving them a glimpse of the whole complicated layered tangled story, right at the beginning, when they are too new to this to listen as doctors, much as they might like to. By the time they're in their third year, they'll be starting to listen as doctors. They'll be a little bit obsessed with the science, which they will probably understand much better than I have any hope of doing, since the genetics and the physiology and the biochemistry and the endocrinology will be so much closer, so much newer, so much more up to date in their minds. They'll be prizing the opportunity to see a rare and interesting disease. They'll be fresh from the classes where they learned to take histories and carry out physicals, and deeply concerned with playing their parts properly as third-year students, trying to take care of patients and impress their preceptors. They will be at home on a hospital ward—or at least, they will be trying to be at home on a hospital ward. They will still be able to feel the tragedy of a parent grieving for a child's illness, of course, but everything will be slightly different, slightly skewed. This is one of their last opportunities to talk to a patient without all of those professional filters, to come in equipped simply with humility and humanity.

Now, I am not telling you this story because I want to suggest that there is something wrong with acquiring those professional filters. I hope and believe that all these students—polite, conscientious, intelligent, hardworking—will go on to honorable and useful careers in medicine, and that they will acquire the vocabularies and the knowledge and the perspectives that they need to be of use to patients and their families.

But there's something peculiar and powerful about standing in the room with them as they listen and look, right now at this moment. It's as if I am seeing a little through their eyes, I suppose, and being reminded how complicated and tragic the world and the ward really can be. It's coming face-to-face with a person behind a diagnosis— even if it's a diagnosis that they haven't studied yet. It's saying—and meaning—all over again that every hospital room, every life, is full of stories more complicated and more tangled than we can ever hope to tease out, but also making the commitment to learn to ask the questions and listen carefully to the answers that may help you understand, at least a little.

Clinical medicine is all about stories. I have been writing down stories about becoming a doctor almost since I started becoming a doctor, and I used to value the exercise in part, I think, because I thought it kept me in touch with my original perspectives. I was telling stories in terms that laypeople could understand, and that proved, didn't it?, that I myself had not been transformed.

That was nonsense. I tell my stories as a doctor now, because I hear stories as a doctor now. I knew the list of interview questions that the first-year students didn't know, and something in me was anxious to fill in the blanks, to ask the details about the little girl's development, or the pregnancy history, or whether there were any children in the extended family who had died in infancy or childhood of any cause. I could have asked my questions, extracted all the information, read up quickly on osteogenesis imperfecta, and come away with a clearly organized medical story, and I could feel myself wanting to do it. Instead, I stood there with the students and I let them make of it what they could.

I asked my son, who is a year ahead of these students, what the second-year students say about working with patients. He told me that since starting medical school, they hear from every side that medicine is not the profession it used to be. Every speaker at every ceremonial moment, he said, feels obligated to tell them that they will not get the kind of respect that doctors used to get, that there will always be HMOs looking over their shoulders, that they will suffer from exorbitant malpractice rates. Well, yes, I said, that's all true. "But then they always say that the most important part cannot be reduced or quantified," he said. "It's the ability to help people, the intimacy, the connection, the degree to which you interact with your individual patients." Well, yes.

At the end, of course, you come back to the whole story, and the whole story is what pulls together all of your medical education. There is the science (and the science is incredibly important), and there is your clinical experience, which teaches you to ask the questions and to listen to the answers, and to listen for what is not said, or for what has not been asked. And there is also your life experience, as a doctor and as a human being. When I stood in the room with the four students and the father and the daughter, what I kept thinking about was what it was like when each of my children was a week old—what it would have been like if I had been home alone with a one-week-old because an older child was hospitalized, away from me, away from the new baby, hospitalized with the worry of a serious diagnosis, with that diagnosis now hanging over the new baby as well . . . So yes, I lied a little when I said I was listening as a doctor. Or better, maybe, to say that I am also a parent, and that being a parent shapes me as a pediatrician, and changes the way I hear other parents' stories.

Becoming a doctor means becoming someone who can ask the questions, understand at least some of the answers, juggle all the stories, and in some way accommodate the emotion. None of these is an easy assignment, and together they are an assignment so complicated that it cannot possibly be done perfectly, no matter how smart, how culturally sensitive, how scientifically well versed you may be. But to believe that it could be done perfectly would be to show your limitations; becoming a doctor, I truly believe, means being willing to exist with the anxieties and uncertainties and complexities of a job that is as big as life.

I liked being in the room with those students because they were awed and moved. I know they probably went in there wanting to be awed and moved, but that's okay. You shouldn't be going into this job if you don't want to be awed and moved. And I saw something else. I saw a generous man, in the midst of his own difficult hospital moment, agree to spend time with a group of first-year students, and open up to them (and then give me permission to write about it). When he almost broke down, the students were slightly embarrassed, but the father wasn't. They were embarrassed for him, I think, worried that he would feel funny about showing such emotion before a group of strangers. He, on the other hand, knew that his emotion was perfectly appropriate, and perhaps he also knew that it was part of what he had to teach them.

So that was the final part of the lesson, and maybe the most important part, and a lesson we all need to learn over and over: this is a very remarkable privilege, this access into people's lives. This gentleman talked to us because he wanted the students to understand what he was going through, he wanted his experience and his daughter's experience to be part of their understanding of medicine. He wanted to tell them that he had had some bad encounters with the medical system, and he wanted to tell them to listen to parents, and to take a second look at children when parents are worried. He wanted to tell them that there are a lot of bad diseases out there which need treatments and cures. And because he wanted to tell them all these things, he was willing to let them into his room, into his afternoon, into his life. And since they will draw much of the rest of their medical training, as we all do, from the kindness of strangers, these students got a hint of both the majesty and the oddity which come with sitting in on the most intense and most dramatic moments in the lives of all these people you don't even know. Of asking them questions and examining their bodies, of teasing out their bodies' chemical and electrical and hormonal secrets, until your memory is stocked with stories and presenting illnesses and differentials and complications, with good outcomes and bad outcomes. Becoming a doctor means accepting your right to ask these questions and hear these stories, and it means giving over to them a big place in your brain and your memory.

I was building toward some kind of peroration in which I would enjoin my students to remember the gratitude we owe the patients who allow us to learn on their bodies and on their stories and on their lives, but I could see that it wasn't necessary. They knew who was their real teacher that day, and they had already said thank you for the privilege. And it occurred to me that the intersection of their own professional trajectories with this "patient encounter" was a rather remarkable moment, and that if I had any sense, I would stop pointing out didactic morals, and concentrate instead on listening to the complicated stories going on around me. The students had entered that zone of the patient's story, and I was privileged as well to have watched them cross the threshold.

THE FAMILY ROOM

Teri Reynolds

There is a golden hour between life and death. If you are
critically injured, you have less than 60 minutes to survive.
You might not die right then; it may be three days or two
weeks later—but something has happened in your body
that is irreparable.

—R.A. COWLEY, MD

When people fall off ladders or roll their cars, get hit by baseball
bats or bitten by hyenas, get shot, stabbed, or strangled, when
their bodies are injured by mechanical force, they are called "trauma
patients." For these patients, it is said, there is a golden hour: a brief
period when even severe traumatic injury can be stabilized with lim-

ited damage to the brain and other organs, an interval after which survival rates plummet.

During my intern year there was one twenty-four-hour period with twenty-three traumas. This is a lot, even for the county hospital. It comes out to nearly one an hour, but since cases are never evenly distributed, some were simultaneous. When this happens, there is an overhead call for the "Backup Trauma Team to the Emergency Department." There is no backup team, but this is a discreet way of asking for all available providers to come to the trauma room. Only once have I heard the operator violate this protocol, when a gunman jumped on top of a car, shot through the roof, and hit all four occupants, including the driver, who somehow managed to drive to the hospital before passing out. Faced with four critical patients and no advance "ring-down" from the field, the operator made a hospital-wide call for "any available surgeon to the Emergency Department—STAT," acknowledging that one time, to anyone listening, that we were not in control.

When the system works, an ambulance medic calls us from the field and delivers the basics over a static-filled radio line: "We've got a fifty-five-year-old man, nonresponsive, BP 110/80, four minutes out . . ." Or they might say, "We've got a twenty-eight-year-old pregnant woman . . ." and lose the line. Thus is the trauma system activated. Doctors and nurses assemble in the trauma room, prepare equipment, don masks, gowns, and gloves, and wait.

Depending on the severity of the injury, the process of confirming the patient's name, birth date, and Social Security number could take much of the golden hour, so to expedite care, trauma patients are assigned a code name under which the initial orders and X-rays are done. This code name is crucial to initial management, since X-rays and other studies cannot be done without a "unique patient identifier," lest we mix up their initial imaging and lab results. Replacing someone's name may seem like adding insult to injury, but in the golden hour, it can be more important to render patients unique than to know exactly who they are.

Trauma names can be any sequence of terms that do not repeat too quickly, and they are themed each year and assigned alphabetically. I don't know who chooses the theme, but this year, we used fruits, and not just Apple, Banana, and Cherry but Jicama, Kiwi, and Lychee. Four years ago, when I was an intern, we used art terms: P was Pastel, O was Ochre, and N was Nuance, which the clerks inevitably misspelled, so that you had to check *nance*, *nunce*, and *nuance* to find a patient's imaging on the computer. Aside from the obscenity of calling a dead man Kiwi, fruits work better.

This all changes, of course, when we leave the trauma bay, trading the chaos of resuscitation for a quiet conversation with family. Some stand as I enter to give news, as if reaching for it, and others duck their heads or fold their hands, as if they could retreat. These are lopsided conversations for so many reasons—the gap between my knowledge and their fear of what has happened, between my day job and their singular event, between the code name and the given one. I never try to explain the fruit or the art to families, and we all try not to use the code names out loud while family are present bedside. Though I've never discussed it with my colleagues, I think we share a tacit superstition that, while the code name is necessary and functional in crisis, to un-name someone in front of family is to put them at risk.

Because I work in a major public trauma center in a city where the rate of gun violence has skyrocketed, the twenty-six letters of the alphabet are nowhere near enough to last a year, so patients are also numbered by order of arrival: Apple-1, Banana-2, Cherry-3 . . . The alphabet, of course, starts over at the twenty-seventh patient, and it is always an index of high volume and bad times when we have two

Apples in the hospital together—when we roll the alphabet from Apple-1 to Zucchini-26, and back around to Apple-27, before Apple-1 is well enough to go home.

I've become inured to rolling over the alphabet, but I still try to pause when we roll over the numbers, to walk out to the ambulance bay and look at something larger, the hills, the sky, when we roll over from 99 to 1. These days there is more time for everything—for teaching, for learning, for reflection, and I try to go to the ambulance bay most shifts, and always at 3 a.m. on a night shift—but my intern year it took almost too much effort to pause for the rollover, to remember what it meant, that a hundred people had been injured so quickly.

The practical learning curve of my intern year ran so steep that it left little room for anything else. The purview of emergency medicine is the beginning of everything, and I actually ran from patient to patient, from floor to floor, from trauma surgery to cardiology to obstetrics, learning and experiencing something new with each task. There was the first time a nurse called me "Doctor" and I didn't look over my shoulder, and the first time I introduced myself by my title. There was the first resuscitation, the first chest tube, the first baby, the first bad news I delivered alone, and my first time declaring a death, which, as it turns out, is more complicated than birth. There will always be firsts, it is the nature of emergency medicine and the reason I chose the field, but the practical aspects—the medications, the procedures, the resuscitation pathways, and how to place hands on a newborn—have become largely automatic. These practical lessons come from experience, but the never-ending lesson of the job is learning to tolerate our own inadequacy in the face of what patients and families experience.

I had an awful series in that year of art: Draw-56, Easel-57, Fig-ure-58—three brothers who'd been shot while walking down the street together. There was a rumor that they were brothers when they rolled in, but no one knew for sure, and we hadn't figured out their names yet in the chaos. Draw had been shot in the chest, but the wound seemed superficial and he looked stable. Easel was shot in the head, dead on arrival. Figure was the one who needed us most—he'd been shot in the abdomen and was hypotensive and fading. We started fluids and blood and sent him up to the OR, where he would die, I found out later. I was the intern on the trauma team and responsible for running the resuscitations and then updating the family, but I couldn't do that until I knew who was who.

The social worker had left to find the family, and my senior resident had rushed Figure upstairs to the OR. I tried the charge nurse, who, for unclear reasons, said she doubted the men were even brothers. The clerk was busy trying to assign an incoming cardiac arrest patient his own code name, and the medics had disappeared to their next call. I turned back into the trauma room, where Draw was lying quietly on his gurney. He was slow enough to respond that I tried my question twice in English and once in Spanish before he answered. He confirmed in quiet but perfect English that they were indeed brothers and that he was the youngest at eighteen. He could tell me his brothers' names, but I couldn't ask him which brother was the dead one—he was pale and glassy-eyed and barely answering my simple questions, so I hadn't told him anything yet, and he hadn't asked.

I went into the next bay, where we'd resuscitated one brother. There was no gurney, and the room that was usually filled with sound, where we were always running into and crowding against each other, felt huge and silent. It was a wreck of blood smears and paper wrappers that we'd peeled off sterile equipment. There was a sneaker in the sink for some reason, and on the wall, a diagram describing the proper position of each player in a trauma resuscitation—trauma nurse to the right, resident to the left. It describes an orderly configuration that I've never seen us achieve and that, given the location of the door, is probably impossible. I found the brothers' sticky black jeans in a ball in the corner and rifled the pockets for ID. I stared at the photographs and tried to memorize what I needed.

Draw, Easel, Figure. Pablo, Cesar, Ramon. Stable, Dead, Guarded. Pablo, Cesar, Ramon. Draw, Easel, Figure. Pablo, Cesar, Ramon.

There's bad news, I thought, and more. I mumbled the rosary of names under my breath as I walked into the family room, a squalid eight-foot square with plastic chairs and peeling paint. I stepped over a plastic Thomas the Tank Engine. Until someone begins to keen or punches the wall, sounds we occasionally hear in the charting room next door, the family room is infinitely quiet. It has different rules than the trauma bay, and the code names that serve us so well in the golden hour mean nothing here. I had to remember what this family called the boys I knew by their unique identifiers.

Pablo, Cesar, Ramon. Draw, Easel, Figure. Stable, Dead, Guarded.

Hello, I said, I'm Dr. Reynolds. A young woman stood up.

This is my mother, she said. The mother did not lift her head.

This is my brother's wife, she said, and my other brother's girlfriend.

I cannot, I thought, screw this up.

I've since been in the family room a hundred times, to give good news and bad, and I'd like to think I'm better at it now. The room has been painted a smooth sea foam green and Thomas the Tank Engine has been joined by a roller coaster for marbles. I have learned some things: to always use the word "dead" when that is what I mean. To make sure that no one is standing and how to catch people as they faint from a chair. I've learned that grief often begins as rage and never to place anyone between me and the door, and that in a small room, you can feel another person's sorrow hit your body in a wave. And I have learned to reassure families that we "did everything we could," as

I tell them with my face that the damage had already been done by the time their loved one arrived, that we had missed the golden hour.

Pablo, Cesar, Ramon. Stable, Dead, Guarded.

Draw, Easel, Figure. Pablo, Cesar, Ramon.

Please, I said, sit. It was my first time in the family room.

ON NOT BECOMING A DOCTOR

Kay Redfield Jamison

When I was six years old, I killed my pet turtle by setting him down on the radiator in my bedroom. It was inadvertent, but he was no less dead for my good intentions. It had been snowing outside and I was certain that the turtle must be cold. If he warmed up a bit, I reasoned, perhaps he would climb to the top of the ramp in his plastic bowl and sleep under the green plastic palm tree wedged into a hole at the end of the ramp. He had never made it to the top before; I thought he would like the view.

It could not have been an easy death, frying on the radiator. I picked up his small body, the shell still hot to the touch, and tried to resuscitate him by dipping his body in and out of cold water from the kitchen tap. When that didn't work, I put him on a plate, took my mother's measuring tape from her sewing box, and wrote down the length and width of his shell and each of his legs in the notebook I kept in a drawer in my bedside table. This notebook contained drawings and measurements I had made of rocks and lizards and tree branches, as well as the paws and whiskers of our cats as they had grown from kittens to cats. After I entered his final dimensions into my notebook, I wrapped him up in one of my mother's lace handkerchiefs and dug a hole for him in our garden. I covered his grave with pansies and holly branches and placed the plastic palm tree on top. He had died. I had killed him.

That winter day, I thought about becoming a doctor. It was not the first time I had thought about it, but it was the first time I took the idea with great seriousness. I was sure that being a doctor was what I wanted to do with my life. I wanted to heal things, to put things right, although my aspirations were never as uncomplicated as simple healing. There was always curiosity involved. There were always the whys and the hows, the why nots? I wanted to heal things, but I also wanted to know why they needed healing. The focus of my desire to heal and my curiosity changed over the years—first it was animals, then the human body, and finally the human mind. But I never seriously questioned becoming a doctor.

It was only years later, when dangerous perturbations in my moods and the writings of William James had shaken my convictions about what I wanted to do with my life, that I set out on a different course. By that time, I had dissected a legion of animals in the basement of our family house and even more in my school and university laboratories. I had fixed, stained, and peered at countless samples of blood and skin, leaves and seeds and butterfly wings, that had caught my interest along the way, and I had become president of the many premed and science clubs that I had helped to set up. I studied chemistry and invertebrate zoology, neurophysiology and psychopharmacology, and added to the growing stack of my notebooks, which were now filled with increasingly detailed drawings and observations from the world around me. Over time, poetry and fragments of plays—generated in different moods and from different kinds of observations—also made it into these notebooks, these fossil records of a scattered but inquisitive mind.

Had I known then what I know now about the pull and the rhythm of moods, I would have noticed that there were weeks when the notebooks seemed to fill of their own accord, thick and inked in many colors, and there were weeks when they lay empty, untouched, irrelevant. These erratic flowings of moods and writings had been part of my life since my first psychotic break during my senior year in high school when, after having flown over the moon with ideas and enthusiasms, a prelude of manias to come, I had fallen into a suicidal depression. It was not until ten years later, after a virulent and psychotic mania, that I was diagnosed and treated for manic-depressive (bipolar) illness, which ran in my family. During the interlude, and for some time after, my moods and academic pursuits lurched wildly about. So too did my certainty that I would become a physician. All of my assumptions had been rattled by my mental instability and newly competing interests.

My errant moods, and the near-ecstatic response I had to reading William James's *The Varieties of Religious Experience*, lured me in the direction of psychology rather than medicine. Looking back, I am quite sure that some of my passionate response to William James was due, at least in part, to one of my innumerable waves of submanic enthusiasm. But, in fact, I felt nearly as passionate about his book in the colder light of normal mood. The expansive subject matter of James's book reflected the expansiveness of his own mind and temperament. It also reflected, as I was to discover later, his personal struggles with mental illness. James was a philosopher, a psychologist, and a physician. He went where his curiosity took him. I was captivated and changed.

I liked the permeable boundaries of James's observations and the tolerant perspective he brought to bear on human nature. Although I loved the idea of practicing medicine, I found that I wanted to study the questions of psychology. They seemed to me to be fundamental to the human condition: Why do we believe what we believe? What is experience? What is normal behavior? When does normal behavior veer into the pathological? Why do moods exist? What role do they play in our actions and in imaginative thought? To what extent do our moods color thinking and, conversely, to what extent does the substance of our thinking affect mood? Why is there so much variation in temperament and in ways of thinking?

These questions spanned widely disparate intellectual and professional territories, as indeed most interesting ideas do. I did not want to be hemmed in by disciplinary boundaries, not when there was so much to take in, so many places in the mind to explore. I liked the romantic, unbounded notion of becoming a doctor of philosophy instead of a doctor of medicine. It seemed less tied to earth and authority.

As I went further in my studies, the unpredictability of my moods and energies cast increasing doubt on the day-to-day practicalities of becoming a doctor. I simply could not imagine sitting still long enough to get through the first two years of medical school. My fluctuating capacity to concentrate and retain new information made the long nights of memorization seem repellant and something I was unlikely to do well enough to survive. Nor was tightly structured learning something I wanted to do. After much reflection, and the kind of regret that accompanies lost childhood dreams, I switched to the graduate study of clinical psychology. I was a duck to water in the freedom afforded by the free structure and long rein of graduate school and never, in subsequent years, have I been sorry about changing fields of study. Psychology remains the source of the questions that most fascinate me, although the world of academic medicine gives me the most conducive intellectual environment and the greatest latitude to pursue my interests. Fortunately, I have found that *not* becoming a doctor allowed me to study and love medicine in a way I could not have done had I actually practiced it.

It was clear that no matter what degree I pursued, I had a restless mind and was subject to intense alternations in moods. These things were a given; my perturbability was not something that was likely to change. I decided to try to make the best of it by learning from those who had similarly restless minds and temperaments. My brother was my original mentor for this. He had crossed intellectual fields willfully and freely, studying philosophy as an undergraduate and aeronautical engineering as a graduate student, and eventually obtaining a PhD in economics. His primary interest is now in public health, but he keeps his early, perhaps purer love for mathematics and astronomy. I watched how he negotiated the world, saw him cross from one intellectual domain into another undeterred by arbitrary academic or professional constraints. It was a good education.

Later, in graduate school, I came across the work of W. H. R. Rivers—physician, medical psychologist, and anthropologist—and I fell under his polymathic spell. I learned from him, as I was to learn from others who bounded from field to field with abandon but discipline, that I should let my mind graze where it wanted to graze. Over time, this intellectual grazing would take me most consistently and most passionately into psychology, medicine, and literature. In each field, I was a participant, and in each field a bit of a stranger.

My clinical and academic interests crystallized after my first episode of psychotic mania. Until then, I had not been particularly interested in studying the pathology of moods, at least not in any systematic way. Once I had recovered from my breakdown, however, courtesy of lithium and an excellent doctor, I became very interested. I read everything I could about the phenomenology, natural course, pathophysiology, and treatment of depression and mania. With a colleague, I established the UCLA Affective Disorders Clinic to treat patients with mood disorders, teach psychiatric residents and psychology interns, and do research into depression and bipolar illness. There is little more motivating in life than the experience of a severe, life-threatening illness, and this alone would have kept my clinical interests focused. But mania and depression are also intrinsically interesting illnesses, ones which are tied not only to death and suffering but to imagination as well. There is nothing straightforward about understanding or treating illnesses so closely bound to the extremes in the human condition.

Clearly, my bipolar illness influenced my academic and clinical work. I brought a marked impatience and passion to what I do and many of the topics I investigate relate to issues raised by my own experience of mental illness. I have focused upon mania as an addictive state, for example, because its addictiveness is central to why so many patients refuse to take the medications prescribed for them, as well as because euphoric states are intrinsically fascinating. I have examined the many other reasons why people do not take their medications, as well as the medical and psychological consequences of nonadherence. Suicide, of course, is the most devastating consequence of untreated or inadequately treated bipolar illness, and I have written about it at length, as well as advocated for its prevention. But I have also written about the positive aspects of the illness, particularly its links to imagination and accomplishment. These links are complicated and incompletely understood, but they make the psychological complexity of manic-depressive illness and its related temperaments all the more intriguing and important.

Not surprisingly, my own illness has influenced the kinds of patients I see, most of whom have bipolar or other depressive illnesses. I have been privy to the terrible psychological pain experienced by my patients and been impressed, time and again, by their resilience, wit, and courage in the midst of suffering. I have listened to my patients as they describe a kind of pain known only to those who have been severely depressed or psychotic, and watched them heal, often far too slowly, and reach out to others who experience the same loneliness, misunderstanding, loss of mind, and loss of innocence. Not everyone who struggles with diseases of mood learns from the adversity, but a remarkable number do. They learn about the transience of their moods and the transience of life, and most of them find a way to give back to others from their experiences. There is nothing romantic about a deadening illness, which can result in suicide, or obliterate through violence or alcohol and drug abuse. But for many, depression and other forms of mental suffering become profound teachers.

No doubt because of my own attempts to derive some use and meaning from my mental illness, I have been particularly interested in the uses to which adversity is put in those who have chosen to be a part of the healing professions. Adversity teaches well, and its lessons are essential to those who heal, whether it is through the practice of medicine or psychology or creation in the arts. Because my entire professional life has been in academic medicine, and because apprenticeship teaching is at the heart of clinical teaching, it has been to young doctors that I have spoken most often about the role of suffering in the making of a compassionate physician. I tell these doctors that medicine is an extraordinary and profoundly human profession. Even in this ridiculously litigious and bureaucratic, mindlessly managed world of ours, medicine is an extraordinary and deeply human endeavor. It is also difficult. Doctors are asked to be scientists, humanists, and healers, and they are asked to do this within the context and constraints of their own lives, temperaments, problems, blessings, and liabilities.

Doctors are asked to diagnose, to treat, to understand, and to heal. They are asked to know science, to know suffering, to know joy, and to understand and address the profundities of psychological and physical experience, human biology, and personality. I talk to young doctors about the inevitable suffering that they themselves will experience, and the suffering they will be called upon to ameliorate in the lives of their patients. I encourage them to read the works of writers who have transformed their suffering into words that inform and heal.

I do this for two reasons. First, I deeply believe that learning from the lives and works of others is one of the most powerful ways of learning. Second, I believe that doctors—like writers—need to draw upon the pain they see in the lives of others and in their own experiences. They need to observe, understand, and then transform the experience of suffering into a more general understanding; this they can use to help their patients and, indeed themselves, deal with what has been dealt them. Sir William Osler, the first physician-in-chief at the Johns Hopkins Hospital, said that "Sorrows and griefs are companions, sure sooner or later to join us on our pilgrimage." This is indisputable. He, like so many physicians before and after him, turned to writers for ways to make sense of grief.

Learning through intense, extreme, and painful experiences, and using what has been learned to add meaning and depth to one's life and work, is a recurring theme in the work of great writers. John Keats, who trained to be a surgeon, wrote, "Do you not see how necessary a world of pains and troubles is to school an intelligence and make it a soul, a place where the heart must feel and suffer in a thousand diverse ways?" This is, of course, a variation on the ancient theme of suffering is learning, of insight as the product of trial and anguish. Doctors, like writers, can derive strength from their struggle to come to terms with pain and adversity, can derive from adversity some redemptive value. Adversity alone does not guarantee good art, a good life, or a good physician. But if it is coupled with imagination, compassion, and discipline, the possibilities for creating sustaining art or a great healer are enhanced.

I have taught for more than twenty years at a great teaching hospital, Johns Hopkins; it has been a privilege. It has been my pleasure to watch good doctors become better ones after their apprenticeships in medicine and life. I revel in the high energy and spirits that accompany clinical and intellectual pursuits, and I see far more idealism than cynicism among my colleagues. I respect my medical and scientific colleagues for their willingness and ability to treat difficult diseases, and for their attempts to understand the underlying genetic, neurobiological, and psychological causes of these diseases. I watch how seriously they take the art and science of medicine. I watch them work long and responsibility-laden hours, fight mindless bureaucracy, and compete against dismayingly smart and energetic colleagues. Most of them feel they are part of a meaningful endeavor and realize their good fortune in their life's work.

Although my work has been that of traditional academic medicine—writing about the clinical features, natural course, and treatment of a particular disease—I have spent long periods of time on the borders of medicine as well. I have found immense satisfaction in this. I am glad I made the decision to become a doctor of philosophy—it has been an unfinished pursuit suited to my temperament—but I have loved the study of medicine in equal measure. I feel blessed in what I do. By choosing a road that took me away from medicine, I find I come back to it time and time again.

MAGIC HANDS

Thomas C. Gibbs

I wanted to see how my hands worked. I wanted to hold an ophthalmoscope, and look into the back of an eye. I wanted to hold an otoscope and look deep into an ear. I wanted to percuss a chest and abdomen and hold a stethoscope as I auscultated the sounds of the body. I wanted to hold a reflex hammer and watch the involuntary movements of arms and legs. I knew I was smart enough. I knew I had the strength to keep going. I wanted to hold the instruments and learn the tricks of the trade right then. I hoped that my hands would work well. Would I be a natural, or would I try over and over? I wanted to practice clinical medicine. And I wanted to do it now.

But first-year medical students don't get to practice medicine. The demands of study occupy all of your time. Still, I wanted to actually see some patients, take a history and do an exam. I was tired of practicing on people paid to act as patients. To protect actual patients from inexperience and harm, access has an order. Patients are admitted to a professor or attending physician, then there are fellows, residents, interns, and finally students. The best I could hope for was standing at the back of the line waiting my turn. But I was older than the other medical students and had been a teacher for several years. I didn't want to wait.

I started looking for opportunities to volunteer in a free clinic. Poor, desperate people with no other options come to these under-staffed, understocked offices open primarily at night. These patients can get away from their service jobs as gardeners and maids only after long days of hard work. The disenfranchised sit and wait. Sometimes it takes all night to be seen; other times the place shuts down as exhausted volunteers head home leaving patients to come back the next day.

I signed up at a clinic where a third-year student I knew said they needed help. I did my first delivery there. I had never even assisted at a delivery before, but a patient arrived in early labor and I was there. The first rule of obstetrics is "do not drop the baby." I delivered the baby, cleared the mucous from her throat, and wiped her dry. I held the baby up and handed her to her mother. I did not drop the baby, but I did fumble the repair. I looked down at my hands. I could see what I needed to do. I saw my hands move the needle holder in and out of the field. Finally, I guided it to the apex of the vaginal lacera-tion. "Stitch, tie, then run and lock," I said to myself as I followed the instructions of the nurse standing over my shoulder. The clinic did not have enough local anesthesia to last long enough for me to finish the repair. There was nothing I could do but keep sewing. "I am sorry," I said. She clutched her crucifix but did not flinch.

"What will you name the baby?" I asked. My patient looked at her baby and said, "Paloma." I asked what that meant in English. The nurse, relieved that I made it through, said, "It means Dove." It had happened so quickly. I wondered if I might have delivered this Dove by sleight of hand, like a magician releasing a white bird from his hat. I looked at my hands and wondered. My patient was happy, it was over. I had finished my first procedure without violating the first rule of medicine: "Do no harm."

I wanted more. I heard of an opportunity in the mountains of Jalisco, Mexico. The Huichol Indians, an indigenous people, live deep in remote areas hidden from civilization. They weave brightly colored yarn into shapes called the Eye of God, the symbol of their spiritual life. They do not speak the language of those who conquered their country. They are withdrawn from others, and the government provides no systematic health system for them.

My contact was a missionary who had established a relationship with a small tribe of Huichol Indians in the Sierra Madre Occidental Mountains. He had crashed three planes trying to get to them. I wasn't sure if he was a pilot who happened to do missionary work on occasion or a missionary who flew a plane when there was no pilot willing to take him where he wanted to go. He made his first connection with this group by rolling oranges downhill toward the Indians keeping their distance. Over the years they became more accustomed to each other, and eventually, the missionary established relationships with remote towns in the area as well.

These people needed medical attention, and anyone who wanted to help was welcome. There would be no departments of radiology, no lab, no referrals. I would be on my own. No one would be standing in front of me, between me and the practice I wanted.

When I arrived at the airport in Guadalajara for a four-day mission, four other students wanting the same opportunity were already there. We shook hands and headed to the plane. It was small and I had my doubts that it could hold us. The Sierra Madres towered in the background. The pilot loaded us up before we could back out. The plane struggled to lift off, and we headed toward the mountains. The warm, humid air currents pushed us down as we neared the top of the first mountain. The pilot banked quickly and tried to circle higher. "Hope we make it next time," he mumbled to himself. It was at this moment that he told us about his crashes. I wondered if he was trying to scare us to Jesus.

On the third try we crossed over the top between two peaks, the other side of the mountain dropping away, and with it, civilization as I knew it. I had no idea what waited for us. The landing strip was an uphill clearing—requiring a slow dive, a last-minute nose-up, and then more speed before we found the ground under us.

The moment the plane touched down, the pilot became a missionary. He showed us to an abandoned adobe hut at the end of the village. "No one will live in it because the Huichols think it is haunted," he explained, "so we get to use it whenever we make a trip." Before I could ask for the story behind this superstition, we were already through the open door, blinking into the darkness, waiting for our eyes to adjust. It was a one-room hut, with an open fireplace, six army cots, and no electricity or running water. I picked a bed, rolled out a sleeping bag, and examined my brand-new medical bag stuffed with brand-new instruments. My equipment looked out of place. I wondered if my medical paraphernalia would be accepted by my patients or if they would think it was a bag of tricks.

We opened the back door to let in light and walked out to check the bathroom facilities. There was no plumbing, but next to the well hung a bucket with holes. This was the shower.

The flight had been nerve-wracking so I decided to clean up. I tested the water—ice-cold. I couldn't get undressed, pull up water, jump under the bucket, and shower before the bucket ran dry, so I asked one of the other medical students to pull up the bucket and hold it over my head. One pailful was enough. I decided I could wait until

I returned to Guadalajara from the long weekend mission to take my next shower.

My first patient was an old woman who, the translator said, couldn't hear. I asked about any injuries. "Her husband beats her when he is drinking," the translator said. Brain injury, I thought. Subdural hematoma (bleeding that forms a clot under the skull resulting in increased pressure on the brain), I thought, as I started my exam. I tested her eyes and then looked in her ears. There, deep inside the canals, stuck in wax, were cotton balls. Apparently when her husband drank he became loud, and the cotton made life more tolerable.

I opened my doctor's bag and rummaged through the instruments. I placed the stethoscope around my neck. I laid the reflex hammer on the table. I found the forceps, and carefully introduced the instrument into the canal and closed it on the wax-impacted cotton. The woman did not move. I pulled gently, then tugged and rotated, freeing the material from her ear.

"Well, there you have it." I said. I took the cotton wads in my hand and showed them to her. She took my hands. "Magic hands," she replied through the translator.

I was suddenly humbled, almost embarrassed, like I had pulled a fast one. Was I someone who flew in on a plane, spent a couple of days, did his magic, and took off? I looked at my hands. Had I just completed a trick like pulling a quarter from behind an ear? I thought about medicine men in tent shows. Was I merely a practicing prestidigitator? Was I someone standing on a platform who knew something, taking advantage of those in the audience who did not? My first patient could hear again. I did not believe I had any magic. Magic is performed at children's birthday parties and in the neon-lit joints of Las Vegas, not here in medical consultation.

Throughout history, we've been called high priest or shaman. But when our incantations turned to science, we became physicians. Now the government has taken even that title away. We are called health care providers. But I was none of these. What I had accomplished required little skill. It had required no training. I was not ready to wear the mantle, the long white coat. I was just lucky.

I left the mountains knowing that I could use my hands and the instruments. There was no need to return. I would find people to help and places to learn without placing my life in the hands of a missionary pilot with a poor flight record.

I returned to school and went back to work in the free clinic. I finished medical school in 1979 and matched for graduate training in obstetrics and gynecology. I began residency. I kept up with the books. I learned protocols and procedures. I did not think about magic.

During my second year at Albert Einstein Medical Center in Philadelphia, I was on the labor floor when a patient in obvious distress was wheeled in. She appeared to be around thirty weeks pregnant. She was accompanied by her mother. Neither of them spoke English well. The translator told me they were recent political/religious refugees from Russia. The Jewish community in Philadelphia had helped them emigrate. She had no prenatal records, and the translator was unable to find out if she had received any care during her pregnancy.

She was wearing a Star of David around her neck. I wondered if the pendant had been a family heirloom worn under many layers of clothes or held hidden in a secret place. Maybe it was a welcome gift from one of the women who helped her find her way to Philadelphia. Could this be the first time she had ever worn it openly? The nurse handed her a plastic bag for valuables and a gown for an exam. I walked out and pulled a curtain between us. I waited for her to lie down on the examination table. When I entered the room, the plastic bag was empty and the star still there around her neck.

I placed monitors on her abdomen, one for the fetal heart rate, one for measuring contractions. I began a complete exam. Her vital signs were normal. There was no fever; her abdomen was not tender between the contractions, so chorioamnionitis (infection inside the uterus) had not yet occurred. I placed a speculum and found bulging membranes filling the vagina. Avoiding a digital exam and possible introduction of bacteria, I rolled the sonogram machine into the room and took a look. Twenty-nine weeks pregnant with hourglass membranes, the cervix open enough to allow the membranes out but not open enough to permit descent of the baby. I estimated the fetal weight to be two pounds. The baby was vertex: headfirst, so we wouldn't have to do a stat section.

I put my patient into deep Trendelenburg position (head down, feet up), hoping gravity would help, and started magnesium sulfate to stop labor. I ordered cultures and blood work. I ordered steroids for fetal lung maturity and hoped for the best. There was no obvious etiology for her premature labor. I presented the patient to the chief resident and the perinatologist. I asked the neo team to come down and talk to her about what she might be facing.

I wondered what she had gone through to get out of Russia, how this might have affected her condition. I wondered how she got from there to here.

I had no personal knowledge of living conditions in Russia. I grew up during the Cold War in Cortland, New York. We had nuclear bomb drills in elementary school. We hid under our desks. My parents talked about digging an underground bomb shelter next to the house; newspaper headlines spoke of spies—theirs and ours. My mother and I stood in a civil defense shack spotting airplanes with binoculars. Mother couldn't identify the planes by name, so she just wrote down and reported the number of engines on each craft. Over the years I had heard stories, I had read the headlines.

But still, I could only imagine what had happened to this woman behind the Iron Curtain.

I hoped we could hold the labor off long enough for the steroids to work. I hoped she would not become infected. But hope, when one is in this condition, rarely holds. Her hope did not last the day. Precipitous labor ensued, and I was called to the room. There was no time for a delivery room, no time for an epidural. I put on gloves and placed my right hand above her rectum and below the vagina. I held my left above the vagina, waiting to deliver the baby. A woman in labor sends her mind to another place when the pain is too much, when she cannot take it any longer. Her eyes do not focus. She cannot hear. Her body lifts up and she pushes.

I delivered a two-pound baby girl. There was no baby warmer, no isolet. The neonatal team had not yet arrived. I cut the cord. I wrapped the baby and held her next to her mother. Arms came around the baby and me. "Magic hands, you have magic hands," she said. I wondered where the words came from. Had they come from her—or me?

The next day, the new grandmother brought me a porcelain figurine from Woolworth's—a Victorian lady with a hat, its bow flying free. Why this gift? What did it have to do with me? It had nothing to do with money, what she could afford, or what she already possessed. Maybe her Russian culture demanded a talismanic gift to someone who had helped her family. Maybe it was some cryptic symbol of what the grandmother hoped her granddaughter would find in America. I will never know.

I am not a hoarder or a collector, but I still have that figurine. Every time we get ready to move, my wife asks me if I am over it yet. I am not over it. I wrap the figurine and place it in the bottom right-hand drawer of the china cabinet with the other good stuff.

I know about my hands. I know that patients want me to examine them, to touch them. They want me to tell them my exam has found the source of their problem. They want to know what it is that I have found, what can be done. They want me to check them every day until they are better, until they are ready to go home.

This time I did not discount my patient's words. I looked at my hands again. The secret of the magic comes from listening to the patient's story, telling me where to look and what to look for. The magic begins when patients give themselves up to me, trusting me. The laying on of hands cannot be taken lightly. There are no cursory exams.

My hands, when I open a patient and introduce them deep into her abdomen and pelvis, can see. I can read with my hands. I feel for the tumor. Before I mobilize and elevate it, before my assistant says, "Look at that," I know that its firm smooth wall is consistent with a benign fibroid. When my fingers sense a rough surface with little cauliflowerlike growths, I know I am contending with ovarian cancer. When my hands move and dark chocolate oozes up, I know there is a ruptured endometrioma, a cyst that causes pain and infertility. Sometimes, when my hand opens an abscess, I can smell the diagnosis. My hands move without thought. They become instruments with a mind of their own. *Clamp, cut, tie, clamp, cut, tie.* The back of my hand holds back the bowel, protecting it. The front of my hand dissects a new plane between a tumor wall and the adherent bladder. I watch the magic.

I know that after I wash my hands and leave the operating room to talk to a patient's family, they will take my hand before I tell them what I found. My hands offer them relief. They have not seen my hands inside the body of their loved one. They have not watched. Still they believe in the hands.

Magic hands. Yes, I have magic hands.

ON WORKING WITH CADAVERS
for cadaver #13

Marion Bishop

L ast week I cut the head off my cadaver. Not in one fell swoop, guillotine-style, but rather, I *dissected her calvarium*: fancy language for cutting through the top half of her skull—from right above her eyebrows in front, to the "occipital protuberance" (that bony bump at the base of your head) in back—with a bone saw.

My lab partners and I had started with a scalpel, carefully slicing a line through her flesh all the way around her head. "Bone saws are for bone, not skin," our instructor had said, and so we diligently cut first. Then one of my partners plugged in the bone saw—a handheld medieval-looking device with a vibrating blade—and around and around our cadaver's skull we went, rolling her from front to back at least three times to make sure we had sawed all the way through her head. We sweated from the strain of lifting, rolling, and holding her dead weight, and formaldehyde and blood from her body seeped into our lab jackets, our clothes, and our skin.

Everywhere, all around us, other students were doing the same thing: the Anatomy lab buzzed with the sound of saws and teams yelling back and forth trying to coordinate their cadavers' next move. At moments, everything seemed to move in slow motion, and tiny rivulets of smoke curled up from each table as saws fought against thick bone. Back at our table, fragments of that bone flew up from our cadaver's forehead and face and into the air. They landed, like ash falling, not just on the table or the floor at my feet, but on my clothes, my hands, my hair, my face, and—when I finally opened my mouth to shout against the sound of the saw—my tongue. Instinctively, I swallowed.

When we were finished sawing, I took out a mallet and a chisel, placed it in the crack the saw had made in my cadaver's head, and began to pound. More rolling back and forth, more pounding, and then suddenly, with one true smack right above her left eyebrow, the skull came free: it popped off all at once, falling back on the table and exposing this woman's naked brain cradled in what was left of her skull.

I held the mallet in one hand and the chisel in the other while my lab partners and I stepped back from the table. We looked at each other and then at our cadaver as though we could not quite believe what we had done. No one said a word, but our cadaver's calvarium rocked back and forth, back and forth, in front of us. Finally, it stopped.

I could not eat lunch that day. The lab had taken longer than expected, and by the time we finished the dissection, sprayed our cadaver with formaldehyde, and cleaned up, the lunch hour was nearly gone. My lab partners and I stumbled into our one o'clock lecture a little late. It had been raining on the walk from the cadaver lab to the lecture hall, and when we got there I was cold and wet. I was also shell-shocked, wobbly; I had not been able to walk a straight line from the parking lot we had to cross to reach our classroom. And even though there was a gnawing in my stomach, I could not imagine what it might mean to eat food. Around me, classmates who had not dissected that day were pulling peanut butter and jelly sandwiches out of plastic bags or munching on hamburgers and fries from the hospital cafeteria. I closed my eyes, put my head down on my desk, and tried very, very hard to listen to what the instructor was saying.

At home that night, my shock continued. I wrapped myself in a ball on the couch, in my bed. In an effort to manage my discomfort, I set aside studying—a huge risk, given the intense pace of med school coursework—and pulled out my favorite coping mechanisms: cooking comfort food, eating ice cream, and walking the dog. When these did not work, I moved on to reading passages from literature I loved and walked the dog, again. My functioning was rudimentary, checked out, subdued.

I have known depression before—and discouragement and despair—but the darkness I experienced that night was something altogether different: trauma. At some point before I went to bed, and after multiple attempts at comfort had failed, I realized I could do nothing but wait to recover—to mark time and try to hold myself together until my soul had a chance to catch up with the actions my body had taken. While I was waiting, I also wrote, telling this story to my journal: "I cut the head off my cadaver today," I explained. "And I am convinced that on some level what I did was wrong, unforgivable, even."

I have always wanted to be a doctor. My father is a physician, and for as long as I can remember, I have wanted to be like him, to do as I saw him do. Some of my happiest childhood memories are of watching him operate—literally and figuratively—as he took care of people in my small hometown. On more than one occasion, I watched television in hospital waiting rooms while he delivered babies or made rounds, and always, I felt somehow important: that inasmuch as the work my father was doing was important, I must be, too.

My first introduction to *gore* came when I was seven or eight years old. There was no full-time emergency coverage in our little town then, and when people were injured or got sick, the best they could do was go to the hospital and ask somebody to call their family doctor. I was with my dad when he answered a call on one of those days, and when we arrived at the emergency room we discovered a boy not much older than me who had somehow been hit in the face with a ball. His parents were distraught, and blood ran out of his mouth, down his chin, and onto his neck. I watched as my father began cleaning this boy up, wiping blood from his bruised face, and comforting him while ascertaining where he needed to be stitched. And then, because it was a Saturday afternoon and the hospital was short-staffed, my father had me wash my hands and put on sterile gloves to help him. I picked up the boy's upper lip, pulled it back toward his nose—exposing the fleshy, bloody underside—and held it in place while my father put stitches in a wound that extended from the top of the boy's inner lip on the far right, across his gumline, and into his teeth on the left.

Although I was short and had to stand on a stool to see our patient, as I held this boy's lip out of my father's way, I felt important. Grown-up. I also felt, for the first time, the kind of subtle dissociation that can come on to make it possible to bear a bloody sight. I had never seen this kind of destruction before—the meaty shards of skin, the bone exposed, the blood surrounding everything, filling up every space it could. I had also never seen the kind of trauma that repair sometimes brings: the stiffening of the boy's body and the tears that rolled down his cheeks as my father injected the anesthetic; the anguished looks on his parents' faces as they held him still; or how each stitch made a fresh new hole in the boy's mouth—a new, smaller wound to heal a larger one—a new crevice for blood to seep out of, and one more puddle for my father to soak up with already very red gauze.

I thought I would faint. Actually, I wasn't old enough to have ever fainted, so I probably thought I would throw up. But in retrospect, I know I was feeling faint, and remember fearing I would lose my footing on the stool, my grip on the boy's lip, and my place at that table.

But I wanted to do my job. I wanted to be there for my father and that boy. I wanted the grown-ups in the room to be proud of me, to believe I had done a good thing. And in spite of myself, I was caught up in the wonder of it all—the beauty of the boy's torn body, the seeming magic of my father's expertise, the sense of being a part of something larger than myself—and I wanted to hang on. I didn't want to be the kid who fell apart. So I bent my locked knees and swallowed my nausea, and I remember very consciously telling myself that everything would be okay—that I could somehow simultaneously witness something that was traumatic and not freak out.

I have been that way ever since. I have attended complicated births of friends' babies, have been the first on the scene of gore-filled accidents, and once even saved a stranger's life by giving him CPR through a sea of blood and vomit in the middle of a New York City sidewalk. And through it all, I have remained calm. Sometimes I have been a little edgy and anxious after the fact, and had a story I needed to tell, but in the thick of the crisis I have remained steady. At some point in my childhood, I learned the virtue of stomaching immediate discomfort and grotesquerie for the greater good of saving a life or simply healing a wound.

I'll admit that I went to medical school, in part, because I liked the feeling of being able to dissociate myself enough from a circumstance to be able to function, to be the unflappable one in a crowd. I also had some gut-level belief that people who were able to make that dissociation ought to do it: that perhaps my quirky psychological accommodations could be put to some good.

But I also came to medical school because on a deeper level I have always been fascinated with people. I spent my twenties teaching English—getting a PhD even—not because of some love of grammar or literature for its own sake but because of what great literature and interacting with students reveal about the human condition. I loved hearing my students' stories and encouraging them to join their narratives to the great narratives of world literature, and I loved what immersion in these stories taught me about life and death and mourning and joy and peace. But at some point the whole exercise seemed too academic and removed from reality to matter very much. I grew tired of reading about death and illness and grief. Instead of communing in a figurative way over the sadness of the human condition, I wanted to place myself in the thick of it: to mourn with those who were mourning, to touch the sick and the weary, and to celebrate with those who were finally free of illness or suffering. I wanted to get dirty. I also had a (probably arrogant) suspicion that my humanities education had somehow prepared me for the trauma of medical school—that the conversations I had been having for years about big life issues would translate into an ability to work in and among those issues with real people. It was a naive assumption.

On the day we cut off my cadaver's calvarium, we also removed her brain. I stood at the head of the lab table with one hand on either side of her brain, my fingers close together and extended up into the remaining part of her face, prying the front of her brain from all of its attachments behind her nose and eyes. One of my partners stood by with a scalpel, and when necessary, we scraped and cut. After forty minutes we had detached everything and so pulled her brain out of the top of her head. My lab partners and I then read the dissector. It told us to turn the brain over and identify all of the cranial nerves. I held her brain in my hands and we did.

My cadaver is a fifty-one-year-old woman. She died on May 11, 2000. Like all of the other cadavers in our lab, she is a volunteer: she gave her body to the medical school before she died. But I do not know her name or how she died. I also do not know if she lived in Salt Lake City, where I now attend school, or if she came to me from far away. But the things I do know about her are peculiar, mundane, and full of meaning I do not know what to do with. She wears a Band-Aid on her left index finger, for example, and her fingernails and toenails are bright red and were carefully manicured before she died. Her arm-pits and legs are also shaved. I like to imagine that this means she found pleasure in taking care of herself, or perhaps, if she was sick right before she died, that someone else lovingly cared for her. She also has no ovaries or uterus, and her appendix has been removed. I try to imagine the health problems that necessitated these surgeries and wonder if she ever had children—and if she did, if they mourn for her, now, or know what I am doing to their mother. I also know that our cadaver has beautiful skin, fine muscle tone, and healthy organs. In fact, she has become a favorite cadaver in the lab: because of her youth and good condition, other students come to our table to examine her and learn.

I also know other facts: that her abdominal aorta—the vessel that carries oxygenated blood from the heart to the gut and all of the organs in the central body cavity—is hard and calcified, and that her lungs and liver are enlarged and heavy. She has broken ribs, and bruises on her chest and its underlying tissues—probably from having received CPR. She ate food right before she died: we found it partially digested when we cut open her stomach.

All of these details speak of her life—and possibly her death—and they seem almost too much to bear. Like a one-night stand that leaves me knowing details about my lover's anatomy, but not his name, I sometimes feel my own humanity—and that of my cadaver—to be lost in the details. The absence of her uterus and the broken ribs speak to a life and death that I am immensely curious about and yet daily am asked to desecrate. It does not seem fair to know a body so well without knowing the life that shaped it. I feel caught in a kind of intimacy that is about knowledge without meaning—about bits and pieces without a whole. I long to tell this woman that to me, she is more than the sum of her parts. But after what I have done to her, I am not sure she would listen.

Struggling with this conflict between the pieces and the whole, on the night after we removed my cadaver's calvarium and brain, I also wrote: "And I am convinced that on some level what we did was wrong . . . or at least that *how* we did it was wrong: hurried, rushed, hacking away at her innocent body to meet the demands of an instructor. A class. Nowhere was this woman's humanity mentioned. Nowhere did the instructor pause to consider what she—or any of the other 25 cadavers in the classroom—had done with their brains. Her personhood, and the use she made of that organ in her life, was never mentioned."

There are names for what we do with our cadaver. I do not like any of them. Mutilation. Molestation. Necrophilia. Cannibalism. Being a medical school student.

There is no argument that we have carved up, carved away, and mutilated my cadaver's body. The scalpel is a tool of discovery whose mark is irreparable. Ten weeks into the job, my cadaver looks nothing like she did when she was alive—or when we first received her. As I write, she sits in six pieces: she is cut in half through her trunk and also lengthwise, her bottom is separated from her top, each limb from the other, and her head has been cleaved in two. Some of this we accomplished with a band saw. The skin that was left has been filleted back, revealing muscle, guts, and bone. Organs are missing—carried off for other people to examine. And although none of my lab partners has purposefully molested our cadaver in the way we usually think of the word, we have followed instructions and placed probes in her vagina, her anus, and her urethra. Sometimes simultaneously. We have sliced through her nipples, cracked open her breasts, and removed all the tissue from her clitoris, leaving it exposed and bare.

Although words like "necrophila" and "cannibalism" seem severe, it is true that I have spent more time in closer proximity to the private parts of my cadaver's body than I ever have with living bodies—except with a lover. I have stretched my body across the length of hers in order to get into the right position to view or dissect different structures. Depending on the day, I have had my face next to her face or genitalia for hours on end, and worn her smell and bodily fluids home in my hair and on my clothes. There is also no denying that I have inhaled and ingested parts of her body: smoke and shards from her bone have burned my nose and throat. And at times, her formaldehyde-soaked body fluids have splashed against my face, and into my eyes and mouth.

I have done all of this in the name of learning and discovery—and with the permission granted to me by my status as a medical school student. But it is a difficult business to perform tasks that in any other context would be considered wrong. Even evil, taboo.

The Anatomy lab after the calvarium and brain dissection was in some ways worse than the actual sawing and cutting. We were to identify all the nerves and holes and cavities ("foramen" and "fossa") of the skull that had been revealed by our dissection. We did this, and at the time I felt very smart, applying names to structures I had not even known existed three days before. But perhaps it was this very naming that was so troubling to me, because although my partners and I hugged each other when we were done, grateful we did not have to come back to the lab for a few days, I left upset.

That afternoon, I visited a group therapy session for adolescent girls in drug and alcohol rehabilitation. As part of medical education, our dean's office has placed students with community agencies to observe and do service. All fall, I have gone every other week to meet with this group. This time, the group leader had asked me to do a presentation on women's health. Some of the girls had had problems with sexually transmitted diseases and unplanned pregnancies. As a representative of the medical community, could I put together a presentation? Something informative and empowering and upbeat?

I could, and did, even full of pictures, diagrams on the board, and anatomically correct language. But partway through the presentation, I noticed a troubled look on one girl's face. She had crossed her legs, wound her arms tightly around herself, and bent over a little: folding up as tightly as she could while still remaining seated. She refused to look at pictures—of her own, female genitalia even—which I had hoped would be helpful and empowering. It occurred to me, suddenly, that she had probably been abused, and that things I was speaking about figuratively, or offering as images, were all too real to her. If so, I was simultaneously recalling the reality of her experience and dismissing it by reducing it to images and words. "What can you teach us about all of this that is true?" I wanted to ask her, knowing my objectification of her experience of being female had not even come close to the mark. But instead, I just toned down my presentation a half a notch, asked her if she was okay, and then tried to remain sensitive to her for the rest of the discussion.

At home that night I wept. I wadded myself into as tight a ball as I could, stayed on the couch, and did not move. I could not bear that I had perpetuated on someone else the same objectification of bodily realities that was being daily foisted on me. I wanted to tell that young woman that she was more than the sum of her parts. Then I wondered whether, if those parts could tell stories, she could be made whole.

I am not the only person who is experiencing the first part of medical school as trauma. All around me, people are falling apart: a handful even refuse to go to the cadaver lab anymore. They want no part of the daily plundering we are doing there. Others fall apart visually or vocally in lab. One student left the calvarium dissection in tears; another screamed and ran out of the room. Many of us refuse to eat meat. Some of the coping mechanisms I see people using scare me. Too many of my classmates have just plain checked out—done the same kind of separation of self-from-reality, action-from-emotion, that I learned as a child, only carried to a much higher degree. They walk around with hooded faces, speaking in anatomically correct language with voices devoid of emotion or even presence. Others have just plain become mean: they lash out at each other, at the dean's office, our instructors, the class officers. Some do not even come to class. That it is trauma we are experiencing is no question. The only question is how we manage it.

And I have gotten all kinds of suggestions about how to deal with the trauma, from people inside the medical profession and out. "Can't you just distance yourself?" both kindly friends and practicing physicians have asked. And "Isn't that kind of distancing necessary, anyway, if you want to be a doctor?" They have advised that I cannot possibly feel this deeply about every body I interact with and stay sane—that some diminution of emotion is essential for success. Others have also suggested that I simply focus on the task at hand and stop worrying about existential issues, or advised that I need to learn to "compartmentalize"—to work on my cadaver with one part of myself while leaving other parts free for emotion and different tasks.

While I hear good intentions and even bits of wisdom in these comments, what these friends and colleagues do not understand is that none of these are coping mechanisms I want to wholly acquire. Although I experienced a kind of pleasure-of-dissociation as a child, the amount of dissociation required to make what I am doing in the cadaver lab tolerable would require a loss of self on some level: a shutting down of the "feeling" part of myself that is the very reason I came to medical school in the first place. And "focus"? On what? The remains of the woman that lie in front of me or the realities that brought her—and me—to this place?

Thinking about this in the cadaver lab, I am reminded of controversial legal work carried out in the 1980s and 1990s by a feminist attorney, Catharine MacKinnon. In *Pornography and Civil Rights*, as well as other texts, MacKinnon argues against pornography by trying to establish a connection between pornography and violence. Specifically—and with pertinence to my experience in the cadaver lab—her definition of pornography includes depiction of subjects' "body parts—including but not limited to vaginas, breasts, or buttocks—exhibited such that [the subjects] are *reduced to those parts*" (italics mine). By extension, because pornography presents the body in bits and pieces, it can lead to a dehumanization of not just the person being viewed but the person doing the viewing. Seeing fragmented images makes us forget the whole. The end result of this, MacKinnon postulates, may even be violence.

Although anatomy labs are a long ways away from legal proceed-

ings regarding pornography, and MacKinnon's theory remains controversial, her suggestion that there may be consequences to viewing
the body in bits and pieces haunts me in the cadaver lab. Although I
personally cannot vouch for a connection between pornography and
violence, I find myself beginning to believe in the dehumanization
aspect of what she describes. Even worse, if *images* of parts cut off from
the whole can cause a kind of desensitization to human experience,
where does that leave me? What does that say about a lonely medical
student doing the cutting?

As part of each anatomy exam, we have a lab practical: two items
on each cadaver are tagged. We walk by each cadaver and have one
minute to name the item before moving on to the next. The last
exam included male and female reproductive organs. There was one
man, excuse me, *cadaver*, in the class who had a very large penis and
immensely swollen testicles because of an illness he suffered right before
he died. "This guy's got gonads the size of Texas," one of the instructors called out on the day we did the genitalia dissection. And indeed,
they were large. When we did a cross section of the penis—scientific
jargon for chopping it off at the shaft—the internal structures were
large and easy to see. For this reason, many students felt sure it would
be tagged for the exam. It was. But as I approached this man's table on
the day of the exam, MacKinnon's words commingled in my head with
all the anatomical terms I had memorized for the test: the instructors
had removed the man's penis from his body, rewrapped the rest of the
body completely in its white shroud, and then perched the penis, alone,
on top of the white lump that was the man's covered body. We had
not only dismembered this man but also hung him out to dry. A most
essential part of his anatomy had been wholly objectified and separated
from the body that sustained it throughout his life.

I know a physician whom I quite like as a person, though he is
a terrible doctor. He is abrupt and dismissive with patients, yells at

nurses and at the hospital staff. And most of this seems to be brought on by a terrible insecurity—an impatience with his own weaknesses that he takes out daily on those around him. I have always figured that this was just his personality, and blamed his parents, a bully in his elementary school, or another trauma from his childhood. Now, I have a different way of seeing him: I cannot help but wonder if at one time he was a kind student, whose good intentions went to hell when he could find no place to keep, or way to hang on to, the humanity he brought with him to medical school.

Recently, someone explained to me that medical schools were based on a military model. And I mean this not just in terms of the brutality or intense pace (the first year of medical school has sometimes been compared to boot camp), but also that medical schools grew out of military needs: war and field hospitals have often been training grounds for physicians and surgeons. Ironically, much of what we know about saving life today has been born of death and conflict. A good example of this is the Hare traction splint, a device used to immobilize the leg when the femur—the large bone in the thigh—is broken. The splint was perfected in World War I and consists of braces, straps, and weights that straighten out the spasming massive thigh muscles and prohibit excessive movement of the broken bones. Before it was invented, soldiers with fractured femurs usually bled to death before reaching the field hospital: jostling and bumping around in the ambulance on the journey from the front line caused broken ends of bone to jab repeatedly into the surrounding muscle and soft tissue and resulted in massive bleeding.

But the unending trauma of military conflict also necessitated a physician who could take it on: absorbing crisis after crisis, treating each patient with unflappable expertise and calm before moving on to the next—and then the next. There was no time for falling apart on the job or attending to one's own emotions when other lives were at stake.

So medical schools were designed to produce this kind of operator: someone who could be counted on to calmly save lives and limbs. If, after the crisis ended, physicians could also exhibit compassion or kindness to their patients, all the better, but the first goal was a very real—and necessary—kind of clinical expertise.

Physicians and educators of this school of thought would no doubt argue that my trauma in the cadaver lab is a necessary part of my education—part of steeling myself to the job I must ultimately do. They are probably right. I suspect, as well, that they might see my emotion as a luxury a good doctor cannot afford—at least not in the middle of a crisis—and maybe even as a detriment to good practice. Perhaps they would simply tell me to quit my bellyaching. But my argument here is not with their end goal—or the necessity of producing physicians capable of handling multiple traumas. We need people in this world trained to perform such tasks. If the childhood pleasure I experienced helping my father is any indicator, I would even like to be one of those people. My only question is if I am required to put my humanity on hold to accomplish that goal, or if there are ways to get there that let me keep my own body and soul intact.

On the day I cut the head off my cadaver, my great-aunt, Pauline Jenson, died. A fun, energetic woman who had helped her husband run a farm and raised five children, she had finally succumbed to cancer after a four-year battle. I loved my great-aunt and grieved for her loss; but I grieved even more for her children, and for my grandmother, who, in losing her sister, had also lost her best friend.

A few days later, attending Pauline's funeral became a way to attend to my own psychological trauma. I knew I needed to see Pauline's dead body—to see a body whole and undefiled and to remember that death need not always be about dismemberment. I was also scared to see her. But as I approached her body in the open casket at the mortuary before the funeral began, I was struck by how beautiful she appeared, how at peace she seemed. And I had to touch her: I put my hands on her hands and ran my fingers across her cheek. "Yes, that seems about right," I thought to myself when I felt her cold, firm skin, "that's what a dead body feels like," and then was troubled by my own new knowledge: death had never been familiar enough before to be used as a benchmark. Prior to working with cadavers, "dead" was simply the thing you were when you were no longer alive.

Letting this all sink in, I walked outside to take a big breath and be alone for a minute. My father followed. "Too goddamn many dead bodies in my life right now," I told my dad when he caught up with me.

"I know," he said, and handed me his handkerchief. Then, later that day, after the funeral and the graveside service, we spoke again. My father asked me what bothered me so much about working with cadavers.

"It's destruction without redemption," I told him. "In some ways, it would be easier to do these things to a living person—if it could somehow save or help them. But this, there is no meaning to this destruction."

My dad was quiet. "The redemption won't come for a long time," he said when he finally spoke. "But eventually, it will add up in the lives this woman's sacrifice allows you to save."

On the day we removed my cadaver's brain, there was a time when I held her upright, sitting, while my lab partners worked on pulling her brain out the back of her skull. It was a strange image, and a strange experience, really: we had not bisected her down the middle yet, so I had my arms around her shoulders and my face next to hers, as if she were ill, and I were helping her sit up in bed to take a drink or adjust her pillows.

It was the day before Halloween. People walked by and made macabre jokes. "It's like *Indiana Jones and the Temple of Doom*," someone said, recalling the moment in the film when Harrison Ford's character eats monkey brains. "We ought to take a picture," other people said. "It's quite a sight, really, especially at this time of year."

But as I held that woman, I grieved for her, and for those twenty or so minutes while my lab partners finished digging her brain out of her head, she was all too real to me. Although I knew she was dead, I somehow imagined that she was there, and that in holding, supporting her in that all-too-human way, I was helping her participate in some strange, maybe even sacred, last rite. I heard lines from Dylan Thomas's poem about resisting and fighting death, "Do not go gentle into that good night," in my head. And I wondered if donating her body, my cadaver, to the medical school had been this woman's way of raging "against the dying of the light." In allowing us to hack her to bits, she was striking one last blow at death—living on in what I had eaten and breathed of her, but also in my lab partners' and my memories of her as well.

This idea, and my father's words about some future redemption, are the only things that bring me any peace. I hold on to them, and try to hear my dad's voice in my head every time I pull on rubber gloves, put on my stained lab jacket, and walk into the Anatomy lab. I run them through my mind as I cradle my cadaver's brain in my hands or wheel her naked body to the band saw for the severing of her next part, and the new cross section of tissues it will reveal.

And although I know she is dead, sometimes I stop in the middle of all this dissection just to touch my cadaver—not as a future physician or someone who holds a scalpel in her other hand, but simply as one human being to another: to hold, to steady, and to comfort. I squeeze her fingers or rest my hand against what remains of her shoulder, her wrist, her forehead. And for some reason, at the end of every dissection, I reassemble her. Like putting back together some giant, human jigsaw puzzle of my own making, I always realign her parts, placing right limbs back on the right side of her body, and left on left, before making sure all her organs are in their appropriate cavities. Finally, before I cover her body in its shroud, I balance her brain in the remaining wedges of her skull and place the bisected sides of her face together again so they meet where they should, at her nose.

In these moments, as the Anatomy lab grows quiet and my work for the day is done, I try to believe that what this woman and I are doing is greater than the both of us: that someday there will be redemption for her desecrated body and for my own tortured acts of desecration.

GOING TO ABILENE

Elissa Ely

I knew a man who became paraplegic after voices commanded him to jump from the top of a building. He did, twice. His voices disappeared—their work was finished—but delusions persisted. In the state hospital, he believed he was being raped continually by nursing staff, who entered his room each night and hypnotized him into quiescence. Sometimes he felt that they assaulted him during the day, even in the very moments he was talking to others. He would grip his wheelchair and shake in the middle of a conversation. He would turn red and blue, like something twisted out of balloons.

There were medical consequences. He caused himself to vomit, which led to malnutrition. He did not allow his catheters to be changed, refused treatment for constant low-grade infections, and wouldn't let nurses near the pressure ulcers on his buttocks that needed debriding. The ulcers were recurrent, the psychosis was treatment-resistant, his behaviors were demanding, and his presence—though it had its reasons—unendurable. Even the most pleasant and demented patient refused to share a room with him. He spent years alone in a room at the end of the hallway.

My patient had a small, beaten-down mother who sent cards to staff on holidays. She visited him faithfully and ferociously, through all variants of psychosis and all variants of psychiatrists. She came to the Team, bringing notes she had taken—books of them after all the years—in order to ask respectful questions about symptoms and medication side effects. She would never have dreamed of telling us our business, even though she was forced to rely on us—the randomly chosen us—to ensure her son's existence. We could hear him at the end of the hall sometimes, screaming at her.

We decided to enlist him into the Team as a formal member. It was an unoriginal strategy, culled from textbooks, meant to be preemptive. Every Monday afternoon at 2 p.m., we would bring him in for a consultation. We explained that we wanted to hear all the details of his experience, but only in as much detail as fifteen minutes would allow. Fifteen minutes was the therapeutic box. In that short time, experiences that overcame him could not overcome us— and we hoped, eventually, somehow, he might not feel so overcome, either.

The news he brought at first was unrelentingly grim: nightly rapes, hypnosis performed upon him by nursing assistants, malignant forces causing him to behave in terrible ways. There was no mercy.

Similar descriptions went on for months, accompanied by demonstrations of chair-gripping and -shaking to assure us of their ferocity. We came to dread our good idea. Then one morning he wheeled himself into Team, pulled up and braked beside the social worker, and leaned over, eyelash to eyelash. His voice was filled with authority. It seemed to be coming from someone else.

"I'm going to Abilene with ten thousand head of cattle," he said, in what I later realized (though I honestly think he did not) was a middling imitation of John Wayne. "Are ya coming with me or not?"

We had heard many shocking requests in Team, but never this. We asked him to repeat it.

"Are ya coming with me or not?" he said.

The social worker, who is an unfazed saint, answered immediately. "I'm coming with you," she said.

He nodded brusquely, and wheeled himself over to the physical therapist.

"I'm going to Abilene. I've got ten thousand head of cattle. Ya with me or not?"

"With ya," the therapist said.

He asked the head nurse. He asked the internist (who was willing to go to Abilene if everyone else was going). He asked the dietician. He asked me. He polled everyone in the room. It was unanimous. He was taking us to Abilene, ten thousand plus.

"That's all I wanted to know," he said, and wheeled himself out.

Slowly, very slowly after that, his delusions began to shift. What caused them to change was a mystery. It was not our preemptive strategy but something deeper and more humane. They were still delusions, but instead of being torturous and self-preoccupied, they blossomed, and became benevolent and grand. He had a task. A large herd of steer and, as it turned out, all mankind were under his care now.

Over the following weeks, he updated us on evolving projects, as they grew increasingly heroic. He needed to divert an asteroid heading toward North America from destroying the country. It was a physically exhausting task but necessary for the safety of the continent. He also arranged for the donation to child welfare charities of millions of dollars earned from writing Hollywood screenplays, as well as after-tax profits of several sports teams he owned (only winning teams). These last obligations were not as taxing as the asteroid diversion. All they took from him, he explained, was money.

There were medical benefits to his altruism. He started shaving, stopped vomiting, and allowed his catheter to be changed. His nutrition improved. Eventually, the wound clinic discharged him. One Tuesday at 2 p.m., he rolled into Team. The consultations had come to feel like meetings he chaired in the board room of his private plane. He looked around at us and said, "I know you think I'm nuts."

Here it was: the green flash, what every psychiatrist dreams of and few have ever seen—schizophrenia overcome, psychosis suspended. He had been shocked into reality. It was a miracle.

His hands were relaxed on the arms of the wheelchair. His face glowed. "You think I'm nuts," he said. "But here's the thing: there are ten of me in the world—the politician, screenwriter, superhero. I can't wait until they come together in one man."

The head nurse wiped her eyes. It was a miracle that had nothing to do with sanity. He was no less schizophrenic. But his psychosis had been transformed into something blessed, full of hope.

A few months after the herd had left for Abilene, his mother came with him to Team. She did not look well at all. She had a tremor, and her ankles were swollen. At the end of the meeting, she tried to rise from her chair, swayed, and fell back again. Something was certainly wrong.

She wiped her eyes. "Why are you crying?" my patient asked, embarrassed, hoisting her up by an elbow. "I am getting weaker," his mother said. "Oh mother," he said, rolling his eyes. Parents can be so dramatic. But she persisted.

"I am getting weaker," she said to us, then nodded toward him. "But *he*—is getting stronger." The balance had finally changed. All these years she had been holding on, waiting to grow weak while he grew strong. When the right generation is rising and the right one falling (as they are meant to do), what happens next is just the natural order. She wasn't weeping. She was rejoicing.

If a man is ready to leave for Abilene, you must gather whatever pots and pans and horses and tack and supplies you can lay hands on at a moment's notice and saddle up. The weak have grown strong; there is miracle in the midst of sickness. Sometimes, we are led by our patients. Humbly, we follow.

SINE QUA NON

Peter D. Kramer

Why did I become a doctor?

Because on an autumn afternoon, the weather was glorious, as it is not always in London. Because I had known I would arrive at my analyst's—Max's—waiting room early and so brought along a small paperback. Because the book was a selection of John Dryden's poetry. Because Max's office sat near Regent's Park. Because given the fine weather and the proximity of a grand lawn in the middle of town, *rus in urbe*, I chose to read outdoors. Because I had ulterior motives, hopes that a young woman, the sort one dreams of meeting in a London park on a sunny day, might spot my Dryden. Because such a young woman did take notice, and because she was Gwendolyn. That's why and how I became a doctor. The mechanics were easy; I took extra science courses, and I applied to medical school. It's the choosing that bears explanation, and we're never good at it.

During the orientation for incoming students, not two years after that unseasonably warm afternoon, a senior physician gave a lecture on humility. There was no illness, he told us, whose cause was known to the fourth level. Or perhaps it was the sixth. The idea was that, yes, we can say that heart attacks are due to oxygen deprivation, which relates to blood vessel narrowing created by plaque, which forms in response to diet and heredity, and so on. But we know embarrassingly little, finally, about the top tier, concerning the nature of cell death, and the bottom, dealing with the translation of genes into consequences. There are problems with the links between levels as well.

It wasn't the number of categories that struck home. Concepts are easy to subdivide; I could, I believe, provide ten tranches of explanation for any number of diseases. But I accepted the greater lesson. We are ignorant, and the difficulty has to do with forms of causation and how they interact. Struggling to explain significant events, we produce fragmentary observations.

My impression is that similar problems arise when we ask how people find a profession. Circumstance plays a role, and experience, and aptitude, and the zeitgeist. But these factors seem insufficient, and they mesh poorly. Nonetheless, here before us is an architect, a teacher, a machinist, a soldier, or, in this case, a psychiatrist.

In scattered paragraphs of my first published book, *Moments of Engagement*, I tried to map out my journey to the profession. In an early chapter, I described a psychoanalysis I underwent in London. A child of immigrants to America, I had just finished college at Harvard, where I had done well enough to earn a scholarship abroad. My successes had brought me scant satisfaction. I remained anxious and intense. And I wasn't pursuing that other calling, the one I had always known was mine: writing. Mightn't I find a less neurotic route toward creative achievement? I entered therapy to see.

Max was an orthodox Freudian given to scrutinizing his patients' word choice. As an undergraduate, I had concentrated in history and literature; psychoanalysis amounted to a practical application of deductive and interpretive skills I had already developed. And then there was the Vietnam War–era student culture, with its ethos that elevated "relevant" callings.

In the final chapter of *Moments*, I demonstrated how these forces merged during a trip I took from England to Israel. In Jerusalem, I met a distant cousin, an elderly Holocaust survivor who had dedicated himself to a painstaking study of philology. After visiting him, I made a mistake on a bus ride and found myself lost in the Negev. In the dramatic fashion common to youth, I imagined dying there and asked myself what I would regret not having accomplished. Under the cousin's influence, I had come to recognize my efforts in academia as superficial. In *Moments*, I wrote: "Like Spinoza, the lens-grinder, like those medieval rabbis who studied practical trades before writing *responsa*, I needed a *handwerk*. Praxis first." My father was a pharmacist. My mother was a clinical school psychologist who in her adolescence had wanted to become a doctor. I would fulfill familial aspirations and become a physician, but of this special breed, those who heal through applying the skills of the People of the Book.

Nothing is wrong with this layering of reasons: family history, current events, societal trends, the personal charisma of Max and my cousin and Sigmund Freud. In passing, in a later book, *Against Depression*, I filled in details about my grandparents' and parents' experiences during and after World War II. That I should emerge sensitive to need in others was not surprising. What should I become except a doctor destined to investigate the intersection of psychotherapy and medication? Although that rhetorical question seems to ignore the problem of how decisions, in fact, get made.

Again: how does a person resolve to become anything? When they, themselves, cannot decide, patients ask this question. One thing leads to another—that route is understandable. But when it's a matter of committing, of applying to a training program, of opting to change direction, of active volition, then the mystery arises. The same holds for marriages, of course. One answer is, you just know. But that "just" requires emotional equipment: enthusiasm, moral passion, resolve, self-confidence, hope. The question becomes: what energizes choice?

That's where Gwendolyn comes in. She had a peaches-and-cream complexion, sparse freckles, and strawberry blond hair verging on red. Her typical facial expression was embarrassment. She was modest or humble on her own behalf, but on yours as well. Looking at her, I often experienced myself as the gross American whose solecisms Gwendolyn might mask by holding up her end. Oh, and she had an impish streak, in the manner of the downtrodden who maintain a reserve of spirit— the ability to twit the oppressor, a category that embraced many men in her life. Gwendolyn was my age, just out of college, though she seemed younger.

We compared reading matter. Hers was Robert Graves, *Goodbye to All That*. Gwendolyn reminded me that Graves derided Dryden, as having "found English poetry brick and left it marble—native brick, imported marble." Did I really like Dryden, or was I merely flourishing a book, to make an impression? It seemed to give Gwendolyn the upper hand that her poet scorned mine, that she was reading about men at war and I about—whatever Dryden's heroic couplets add up to. I was, I should say, in an earnest stage, trying to fill gaps in my education. I had a feel for eighteenth-century verse and wanted to reach backward. Gwendolyn laughed at me, for my boldness in staring at women, for my presumption in thinking she might find me interesting.

She possessed, I should say, a cupid's-bow upper lip and impossibly pale, translucent skin on her neck above the collarbone. Her figure was at once boyish and promising. Years later, seeing Gwyneth Paltrow in a breeches role in *Shakespeare in Love,* I thought of Gwendolyn.

That warm afternoon: I needed to leave. I had an appointment with my analyst. My farewell intrigued Gwendolyn. We might meet again after all, perhaps in two days time, an hour earlier, at this spot, weather permitting.

I said, "It may be fine—I expect it will be fine." The echo of Virginia Woolf earned me a half smile. That I was not utterly unread reassured Gwendolyn.

That I was a bit of a priss and a prig was the subject matter of the analysis. So was the pursuit of women.

I adored Gwendolyn. Of American authors, her favorite was Saul Bellow. By her account, her rural, Methodist relatives resembled his urban, Jewish characters. With my brashness, I might well be one of those.

But Gwendolyn did not trust me, not as a lover. She was fragile, recently recovered from a long interval of anorexia and still in treatment. As if to protect herself, she became fast buddies with a socially awkward friend of mine. They shared intimate jokes, went to the cinema. With me, Gwendolyn discussed literature and psychiatry. She began to tell her story, as if I were a natural repository for shameful secrets.

She had been self-destructive, for subtle and obscure reasons, a cutter, suicidal. She told tales of country life. Her family owned orchards and a cider mill. Rats really did live in the barrels. Gwendolyn would share disgusting thoughts, to see if they would push me away.

In college, I had known another girl who suffered anorexia. The condition was less common then, but there was enough around that you could not go the four years without encountering it. My classmate had been quite disturbed. Schizophrenia was at issue, or some other terrible affliction, beneath the eating problems. She had commanded my loyalty, this college girl, as someone injured who required company. But she had scared me as well. She could be fierce—or simply unreachable on a given day.

A paranoid man gravitated to my Harvard House, lurked, accosted undergraduates. A classmate threatened me physically and then, over a semester break, committed suicide.

Gwendolyn gave a fresh face to mental illness. Imagine listening to her daily, in the fashion of Max with me. Heal her, hold her—how different were these wishes?

Gwendolyn asked that I listen, as the price of flirtation.

I envisaged Gwendolyn in therapy. She would offer her virginal front, denying the sexual impulses that Freudian theory deemed the great motivators. I would be just the man to see past her facade.

To be helpful, to be attentive—these were safe stances, ones that hark back to that childhood among the displaced. Was there also a measure of sadism in my feelings for Gwendolyn? A Freudian would say so. Doubtless Max did. Mooning signals hidden aggression. No, we must mistrust my tenderness; I mean to say precisely that. Perversion energizes sexuality, which then becomes the motive force for—anything, according to Freud. In this case, for imagining myself a psychiatrist.

The issue is not whether I, as I was then, would have made a good doctor for Gwendolyn. I was immature. The issue is what she did for me. The legitimacy and illegitimacy of my wishes—those are what I mean to point to, as elements in the multilayered answer to the question, how one chooses.

In a sense, there was nothing to my relationship with Gwendolyn. I met another young woman. We dated. Together, the girlfriend and I moved into an antique row house facing a small green in Highbury, an extraordinary find. On one side, our neighbor was the groundskeeper for Arsenal F.C.; on the other, Sir Colin Davis, the conductor, known to intimates as "Woolly." Gwendolyn visited, but not often, and then less and less. If she was virginal, still she might prefer to be desired, and I had turned my attentions elsewhere.

I left for Israel. I returned. I spoke with Max about nurturance and aggression, about service and ambition. I determined to apply to medical school. To my daytime studies in philosophy and literature, I added an evening physics course at a workingman's college.

When people wonder how anyone decides, often their complaint is not obsessionality but anhedonia. Nothing grabs them. For those who cannot move because they cannot be moved, I wish—what?—a motive force, which may be to say, a smidgeon of lust.

"How did you become . . . ?" We list the four or six levels and tell the related story: the predisposition, the misfortune, the redemption, the inspiration. To quote Dryden out of context: "Plots, true or false, are necessary things." We do not mention Gwendolyn. We know that if we do, our motives will forever be deemed suspect. Even now are we free of warped desire? For years in training we psychiatrists work on recognizing and corralling countertransference, achieving what straightforwardness we can. We use the word "sublimation," referring to an outdated formulation, concerning the transformation of libido into productive work. Still, about Gwendolyn we are silent—but is she not, to allude to another favorite poet, the "without-which-nothing of pre-eminence"?

On my shelf, I find *Pope*, in the Laurel Poetry Series by Dell, a thin, sepia-toned paperback, thirty-five cents. I see that Reuben Brower, who taught me Yeats sophomore year, edited *Dryden*, which may be why I picked up that volume after college. It appears to have gone missing. Odd, that in my decision making, poetry should have played a prominent part. Perhaps it was a cowardly act to have chosen medicine when I so loved literature. I see that for me this question, about becoming a doctor, hides and reveals a second: how does one become a writer?

THE DOCTOR IN MIDDLE AGE

Charles Bardes

1. THE DOCTOR IN MIDDLE AGE

The young physician, fresh out of medical school and residency, bristles with science. The latest biology, the newest medications, the hottest studies, all lie ready at his fingertips. Patients and colleagues alike marvel at his sparkling aptitude.

Twenty years pass, and the young physician is middle-aged. His science, unless he is himself a scientist, is not so fresh. What then?

The ancient theory of the climacterics held that a man's life is divided into stages, each seven years in duration. (Seven, of course, is a magic, sacred, and symbolic number: the seven heavenly bodies, the seven seals, the seven-league boots, the seven sages of antiquity.) At seven years he becomes a page, at fourteen a squire, at twenty-one a knight, and so on. A modern remnant of this belief is the age of majority, twenty-one years. In this system, the perfection of life is age forty-nine, seven times seven, the magic number squared, the time when a man's talents have all developed but have not yet begun to decline, his apogee on earth.

Classical medical theory also gave a special province to middle age. As the Roman encyclopedist Celsus writes in *De Medicina* (II.5), "But middle age is the safest, for it is annoyed neither by the heat of youth nor the chill of old age. Old age suffers from chronic diseases, youth from acute ones."

The young doctor is shocked by infirmity and death, but the patients who suffer these do not resemble him. He feels sympathy but not affinity. Twenty years later, it is the patients quite like himself who must be diagnosed and medicated, who sicken, suffer, and die.

The physician in middle age worries about his obsolescence, panics a little, knows less than he ought, forgetting much, stumbling in the new disciplines. He offers not the science of his youth, nor the wisdom of his looming old age, but maybe something that partakes of both, a sort of informed kindness, knowing enough not to be merely kind, and kind enough not to be merely knowing.

2. DEMOCEDES THE PHYSICIAN

Herodotus tells the story: how Darius of Persia, absolute ruler of half the known world, had injured his ankle dismounting a horse. Days passed and the pain grew worse, despite the best efforts of his Egyptian doctors. He summoned a prisoner of war, Democedes, a renowned Greek physician who had hidden himself among the slaves, dressed in rags. Threatened with torture, the physician treated the tyrant, who rewarded him with two sets of gold fetters—which led Democedes to ask if the king meant to double his sufferings in return for his care.

The physician's reward, the physician's bondage—two serpents, two chains, one and inseparable.

3. Gentle hero

Doctors are big shots. In high school and college, they were near the top of the class. In medical training, they come to master— more or less—a powerful technology for treating disease. Once in practice, they assume a privileged role in society: well paid, respected, and entitled. They park their cars in spots where anyone else would get a ticket. Small wonder that doctors so often feel themselves to stand atop a hierarchy, one that extends within and without medicine. The hazards of such a position are pride, ego-tism, vainglory, self-aggrandizement, and all the other expressions of me-centeredness.

But in providing medical care, the doctor is often called to a much humbler role. Quietly listening as the patient speaks of defecation, secretions, body functions; suppressing exasperation as the patient spins out endless circumstantial details on the one hand, and omits the main issues on the other; holding the sick person's hand by a hospital bed; filling out forms.

The Greek poet Pindar, in his Third Pythian Ode, names Asklepios, the mythological hero-god of medicine:

> *the gentle craftsman for the limbs of men,*
> *hero for all who suffer from disease.*

This seems to imagine the opposite of personal hubris or me-ness. One wonders if the gentle hero would qualify for admission to an American medical school these days.

4. INURE

A twenty-one-year-old man, considering a career in medicine, visits his onetime pediatrician to discuss the profession. He wants to know something very particular: how does the physician face his patients' suffering without hardening his own heart, how does he engage their pain without inuring himself against the very experience he seeks?

The doctor responds with a story, how he had to tell a mother that her eight-year-old son had drowned in the backyard swimming pool. It was hard, is all he can say, it was very hard, as he looks away.

The collegian remembers the pediatrician as tall, upright, square-jawed, admirable, manly. He was strong, he sailed on weekends, he wore a blue-and-white seersucker suit in summer. He lived in a stone house with a stone garage, gray pewtery fieldstone. In the family mythos, he never made mistakes; it was his substitute, one unfortunate day, who had missed a sister's appendicitis and allowed it to rupture.

Now, fifteen years later, the pediatrician has changed. His posture is stooped. His upper back bends forward. He sucks incessantly on peppermints, like a chain smoker, making little smacking and slurping sounds. He seems distracted. His bow tie, it seems, is frayed.

5. MAGDA

A forty-seven-year-old woman, the mother of twins, visits me because of abdominal pain that began two days ago. When examined, she appears to have an obstruction of her large intestine. This situation is unusual and potentially severe, not only because an obstructed intestine can burst, with catastrophic results, but also because the possible causes of obstruction include some very serious conditions.

We rush her to the hospital's emergency room. A CT scan confirms that the intestine is obstructed by a mass in the colon—this makes cancer all the more likely. She goes to surgery that same night. The surgeon's findings: intestinal obstruction due to a mass, which proves to be not cancer but—endometriosis. This benign condition occurs when tissue ordinarily lining the inner surface of the uterus becomes implanted elsewhere in the pelvis. Though the patient must undergo major surgery, she will be fine.

What was the doctor feeling, while all this was happening? My first emotion was concern for her—someone I liked was in danger. My second was worry that I had overlooked something in the past, and I reviewed her records to see if this were so (it seemed not). My third was also worry: would the system work properly (it was late Friday afternoon), would she get appropriate care from the doctors I needed to help me? My fourth emotion was fear: was this cancer, would she recover?

My fifth emotion was *happiness*, when I learned that she was all right. I gleefully told the story to some students of mine who happened to be at the nurses' station. I called my wife to share the news. I remain happy as I write these lines.

What strikes me as noteworthy is that my sequence of emotions encodes a crucial distinction between medicine and science. Medicine *wants* something. Specifically, medicine wants the patient to do well, to have a good outcome. Science, at least in principle, wants nothing and is indifferent to outcome. Galileo should not be happy or sad if the heavier ball falls faster than the lighter ball, or vice versa; he cares about observing closely, and interpreting the facts. But the doctor wills something, wills good for others; and this goodwill, this benevolence, is our profession's deepest core and truest guide.

6. Revolving door

Every patient has one main doctor, but every doctor has many patients. This paradox affronts the patient, who somehow would be the *only* one. The patient who sees another leave the consultation room, just before he himself enters, often drops a comment, also a commentary, also a critique. "Next!" he might say, or "Well, a real revolving door!" The physician hears these remarks almost daily.

The relation between the patient and the doctor: individual, intimate, concentrated, benevolent. The two, for their minutes together, focus entirely on the issue at hand, which is the well-being of the patient. How, feels the patient, could the doctor have another?

We use the one word, "love," to mean so many different things. Love between lovers, between spouses, between two who are betrothed, is exclusive; each loves only the other. Love among family members is inclusive; the parent loves the child but may have several children, and loves them all. The child, meanwhile, faces perplexity: is the parent only my own, or must I share with these interlopers who are (they say) my brothers and sisters?

The patient faces the same perplexity: is the doctor only my own, or must I share? How dare others demand his attention? How dare he bestow it? How dare the physician love another? How dare the physician hurry?

And so the patient signals his protest: revolving door, I mean nothing to you, it is all in-and-out, one following another, treacherous libertine, falseheart. The Duke in Verdi's *Rigoletto: Questa o quella*, he sings. *This one or that one, they're all the same.* Mozart's Leporello: *Ma in Espagna, son già mille e tre*, sings the servant. *But in Spain, already a thousand and three.*

My office is my own—a desk, a computer, bookcases, books, diplomas, art on the walls, family photographs, certain keepsakes. There are two examination rooms across the hall; these I share, these are functional, these are nearly anonymous. The patient in the exam room wears an anonymous pajama, then reclaims his own clothing to meet me in my office. There we talk. There we sound and resound our intimacy. How could you love another? And if you do: perhaps I shall lay you low.

7. Two doctors

Two doctors meet at the nurses' station. They begin to talk about a patient who has just suffered a heart attack during bypass surgery. Was the surgery indicated? Necessary? Beneficial? What was the evidence that supported the decision to operate?

One, a senior cardiologist, continues unexpectedly by relating a phone call from a woman, recently widowed: "You don't remember me, but six months ago you advised my husband not to have heart bypass surgery. You said that, because of his leukemia, he would survive the operation but not the hospitalization, that he would get infections and dwindle in the ICU and then die in the hospital. You said we should take him home. And that's what we did, and we had six wonderful months together, Christmas and then Easter, and then he died of his leukemia. I want to thank you."

Why does the cardiologist relate this tender story? It places him in a favorable light, of course, but this particular man has better things to do than to boast. More important, the tale serves as a reminder that the caring physician must restrain the forces of technology as well as administer them.

Most important, he was telling his slightly younger colleague about the different ways doctors *know*. Best recognized is the application of science. The physician knows biology, chemistry, and physiology, knows how they work in the human body, knows the results of clinical studies that argue for or against a given therapy. Less recognized, but equally important, is a second way of knowing: the physician accumulates stories, layer upon layer. A few stories make only for isolated anecdotes. But the thousand stories of an experienced physician make a book, and the hundred thousand stories he has heard make a library, a vast accretion of personal and collective knowledge. The science is important, of course; but the stories too are important, and without them we know only halfway, and the leukemic patient goes to surgery, and dwindles in the ICU, and dies in the hospital sometime in late November.

8. THE WARDS

At a teaching hospital, the doctors take turns as the attending physician on the wards. For one or two months a year, each serves as the doctor, supervising interns and residents, for people who arrive at the hospital without a physician of their own.

It is a spectacle from hell, a vision of shades, a procession from Tartarus, God's own outcasts.

Some of the patients are travelers who land unexpectedly at the hospital with chest pain or the like. Others, from nearer homes, come by the ambulance driver's whim or exigency. Most, however, come to the emergency department out of a profound disconnect from the usual bonds that provide for medical care.

Every night brings an alcoholic or two, in various stages of delirium tremens. Our job is to prevent their seizures, to cool them off for a week or so, to offer rehabilitation, to acknowledge their promises for reform—like the youthful Augustine, *Lord, make me virtuous . . . but not yet!*—then discharge them, only to meet them again a week or a month or a year later. Each day a transfer from the nursing home, always with an infection, whether in the lung or the urine or the skin. God or Nature beckons them home and we the doctors interrupt the call, stave off death for a later day, another pneumonia, another ghastly infection. Especially among the homeless and the very obese, infections of the feet and legs are particularly frequent. The story repeats itself: antibiotics, rest, release from the hospital, return a few weeks later.

The screams may be heard along the corridor: "I need my pain medicine!" What they mean is narcotic: morphine, and its close relatives hydromorphone or oxycodone. These are not the patients with cancer, who call for help gently. Those who scream seem to be wired differently, as though pain, even a little pain, brought unbearable mortal anguish. There is no comforting them, only a narcotized haziness, a transient satiation of some unknown neurologic receptor, until a few hours bring the cycle round again. A few are faking their illnesses, just to get the narcotic, and it takes the doctors a day or two of unpleasant suspicion to confirm the lie.

A diabetic with uncontrolled glucose elevation, whose glucose levels will never be controlled because he has no intention of controlling them. A hapless woman with cancer. Paralytics—gunshot wounds, gangland retributions, seem to be the commonest causes—with skin that can never be made whole. Manipulators who know that a complaint of chest pain will always earn a night or two in a warm bed.

Medicine at its best invokes a kind of therapeutic libido, a shared desire, in which the patient wants to get better and the doctor wants the patient to get better. Not so here on the wards, all too often a place not of hope and victory but of despondence and defeat, not of trust but of mutual suspicion, not of tenderness but of officious management, abasement on all sides.

The middle-aged doctor who serves as attending physician on the wards revisits his own internship, twenty years past, feels again the old traumas, the old complicities, the wounds he inflicted, the terrible acts committed in the names of Apollo the Physician, and Asklepios, and Hygeia, and Panacea.

An island of many Crusoes, some wracked by storm, some by the vindictive blow of an unsupplicated god, some by their own incompetent seamanship, some by malice. The young and earnest doctors, en route to something they imagine better, a distant sail, a footprint in the sand.

9. Aggress

Medical talk often uses the term "aggressive" to indicate vigorous, emphatic treatment. The word can be used in a positive or a negative sense. A doctor may promise to be aggressive, implying that he or she will make every effort to deliver effective care. Or, doctors may be criticized for not being aggressive enough—in treating high blood pressure, in dosing chemotherapy, and so on.

But why should the physician be aggressive at all? The term implies assault or quarrel. It derives from the Latin word for "attack." Later in the word's etymologic history, it comes to signify forcefulness or assertiveness, its pugnacious tone reduced but not erased.

The aggressive physician will fight the disease, and by forceful means. One imagines fisticuffs, weapons, blows being struck. But the patient—from the Latin *pati*, to suffer, to endure, to be acted upon—is a person, a sentient being, bearing the brunt of the attack. Perhaps the unaggressive physician, letting the blood pressure stand a little higher than "ideal," reducing the chemotherapy dose after the patient develops side effects, is merely trying to soften the blows. Or, more radically, to foreswear attacking the patient at all.

10. I WANT IT TO GO AWAY

A fifty-year-old man falls and injures his shoulder. It hurts that night, and again the next, and again when he lifts something or moves a certain way. What does he want? you may ask him. *I want it to go away.*

For children who are injured, the hurt does go away, most of the time. Children heal quickly. Sprains, twists, and cuts are soon gone and soon forgotten. In early and middle adulthood, the injuries take longer, the pain lingers. For most injuries, the rational patient would wait a few days to see how things go, then see a physician if there were no improvement. The visit would lead to antiinflammatory medications, X-rays, perhaps an MRI, perhaps a subspecialist consultation, perhaps physical therapy.

But that's not what I want—I want it to go away. The adult patient who stays home, hoping against hope that the hurt will disappear, returns to the mind of the child, whose world is one of magic. Only in magic do things disappear of their own. Indeed, the entire medical world of the child is one of magic. The wound disappears by itself; or I see a doctor and submit to his rituals, his secret gestures, his incantations, his hocus-pocus; he makes the sickness go away. Penicillin might as well be a pentagram, the prescription a charm, polio vaccine an enchanted elixir. We slurp it down, it tastes sweet, the nurse and the mother make glad.

The adult finds that his injuries do not disappear so quickly; they stay awhile, or perhaps they stay forever. The magic is gone, the sage is a technocrat, the nymphs are departed, the dryads are nothing, the rocks and trees are only that.

11. NORMAN

He called every week, sometimes twice. Seventy-eight years old, and still working in finance, whether productively or marginally I never knew, he produced symptoms, new or old, at an alarming rate. He felt phlegm in his throat, he felt chest congestion, he felt a lump in his throat, his skin itched, his ankles were swollen. His wife, herself chronically ill but avowedly stoical, tolerated his complaints with irritated fortitude.

Some of the symptoms could be readily dismissed. Throat phlegm hardly seemed important. Chest congestion, when it had been established that there was no fever, no cough, no chest pain, no shortness of breath, was equally dismissible. The lump in the throat probably represented *globus hystericus*, a sensation described since ancient times, in which one feels the throat constrict as a response to stress. Itching and rash were more problematic: could this be a medication allergy, or simply dry skin, or a dermal response to compulsive scratching? (Observe: no rash in the middle of the back, where a scratcher can't reach.) Ankle swelling: that could reflect something as important as malfunctions in the heart, liver, or kidneys, or as trivial as varicose veins. A few tests ruled out the serious causes.

One day he related a sickness that had sent him home from work. "Sylvie had to wrap me up with blankets, just the way my mother used to do." *Ecco*—the long-awaited key to Norman and his symptoms, to Norman and his suffering. For suffer he did, as irritating as it was to his caregivers. It was Mama and the blanket.

12. Physician absent

The art historian Edgar Wind relates an anecdote about the opening of the National Gallery of Art in Washington in 1941. President Roosevelt spoke, but he addressed not the company assembled before him but rather the radio microphone. Those physically present in the room were eavesdroppers to the real event, which was the live public broadcast.

In the same way, the contemporary physician speaks not to the patient but to those who listen unseen at the other end of the clinical microphone. This phenomenon is most apparent in the doctor's note. No longer a notebook, a place to recall one's observations, impressions, and interpretations, the doctor's note now functions less as a clinical record than as a ship's log for future examiners, the insurers, billing supervisors, lawyers, and searchers after fraud.

The auditor, one recalls, is a *listener*. So too is an audience.

The private note as a form of public speaking is fine when the clinical matter is simple: "The patient had abdominal pain for 2 days. I found tenderness in the right lower portion of her abdomen. I removed her appendix, which was acutely inflamed, and she recovered." It works less well when the matter is complex: "The patient had abdominal pain, off and on, for several years. The examination was normal. Perhaps she has been abused . . ."—for nearly half the women with otherwise undiagnosed abdominal pain have been the victims of domestic violence. The doctor who dares record the suggestion of abuse might well question who beside himself will read the hunch: the various forms of chart police, the patient herself?

The physician speaking to the absent auditors stops talking with the patient who is present. He becomes an abstraction before a microphone. For the patient it is a secret microphone, as if hidden in the boutonniere, transmitting the words that appear to be a conversation but rather simulate one, the monologue of a talking head, the way an orator speaks to no one but a hypothetical posterity. Those present are absent, and those absent are present.

13. PNEUMA

Pneuma is breath, pneuma is wind, pneuma is air, pneuma is spirit, pneuma is the Spirit of God that moves upon the face of the waters.

Against pneuma stands pneumonia, the disease, the killer, the demon, the enemy, the old man's friend. For so pneumonia was called for century upon century, gentle escort to a quiet, quick death.

No man can live without pneuma. When breathing fails, life ends. The ancients marked the end of life not when the heart stopped beating, as we do now, but when breathing ceased; an ear placed on the still chest, a mirror held to the nose. It does not fog, the man is gone. A flame bereft of air shall flicker and end. So shall a mouse in a glass jar.

The breath stops, the spirit escapes, these two events are one.

Modern pneuma is pneumatic, a drill, a tire, a mechanical bird.

Pneuma, for Aristotle, transmitted soul to the fetus not yet born.

A DOCTOR OF NONE

Zaldy S. Tan

"I am wearing polka-dot boxers today," said Kyle Thorndike with a smirk revealing teeth as straight and white as piano keys.

The other twenty students let out short, nervous chuckles, except for the poker-faced Jennifer Stein, who sat next to Kyle and was the next in line to speak. My instruction to the second-year medical students gathered in the drab basement room of the hospital had been this: Introduce yourself by saying something that nobody else in the room knows. After the first grueling year of medical school, the students already knew each other quite well, bonding in lecture halls and tutorial rooms, Facebook wall posts and weekend parties. Over the years, I have found this a good way to break the icy gloss of competitive anxiety that the students come with on the first day of class.

"TMI," hollered Cathy, who had just revealed that she was allergic to peanuts. Everyone laughed some more.

There's about a fifteen-year age spread between my students and me, but their lingo had somehow seeped into my vocabulary, from TMI (too much information) to PIA (pain in ass) and KISS (keep it simple, stupid). In the next nine months they will have to learn mine: AMI (acute myocardial infarction), DDX (differential diagnoses), QOD (every other day), WBAT (weight bearing as tolerated).

The laughter slowly died and the class's attention descended on Jennifer.

"Let's see," she began in a deep, leathery voice. "I used to dive and I was part of the national team that competed in Sydney in 2000. I majored in molecular biology at Stanford, spent a year at NIH to do research in cell signaling pathways . . ."

Listening with half my mind to Jennifer's treatise of accomplishments, I scanned the young faces before me and wondered what novel paths they would carve with those razor-sharp minds brimming with ambition and idealism, the mental sarcasm yet to creep in. Sure, they all seemed eager enough, but a part of me wondered how many of them truly wanted to learn pathophysiology and physical diagnosis, and how many considered my class only as a necessary nuisance, a way station along the path to the most lucrative specialties in medicine. I knew all too well that during the first year of medical school, as they traced the aorta's course from the heart to its tributaries in the brain, they gleaned from their senior peers that the ROAD (radiology, ophthalmology, anesthesiology, dermatology) was the straightest path to paying off their medical school debt, a nice house in an upscale town, private school for the kids, and eventually a comfortable, early retirement.

Not too long ago, I was among them, an ambitious overachiever poised to go into a prestigious, high-return-on-investment specialty, perhaps oncology or cardiology. That is, until one summer when I turned my back on all that I had worked hard for and everything I felt I was due.

On a breezy, blustery August morning ten years ago, I flew home to Pasadena from Providence for the first time in a year. It was a strange homecoming of sorts; the previous night had been the last of my medical internship, that rite of passage that transforms medical student into physician. After a year marked by thirty-six-hour calls and marginally edible hospital food, I was glad to be back home—the first doctor in my family—and basking in my parents' admiration. I feasted on homemade wontons and adobo, as I told embellished tales of my medical exploits. After lunch I lounged in the backyard on my favorite hammock, as turquoise hummingbirds buzzed by and the warm Santa Ana winds lulled me to sleep. I was in that idyllic, postprandial state far away from the stress of the hospital when my mother called my name. Grudgingly, I left the hammock and walked back toward the house.

Half an hour later, I was standing in front of my uncle Pablo's expansive house in Arcadia. On the car ride over, my mother informed me that to make more money my uncle had turned his house into an old folks' home, a board-and-care facility that provided care to half a dozen elderly people with disabilities that precluded them from living at home. A brown-skinned, dwarfish attendant opened the door for us and gave a shallow bow as we entered. My mother shuttled me through what had once been the living room but now served as a lobby, past artificial plants and a not-so-grand-looking baby grand piano, past a couple of cotton-haired women in wheelchairs, and through a long, sterile hallway redolent with disability and desperation.

At the end of the hallway, in what must have once been the master suite, lay my grandmother, Celedonia Marcelo. Above the bed hung a still life of a beach scene and a bunch of yellow lilies in a clear glass vase sat on the nightstand. Through the sprays of sunlight filtering through the curtains, I saw that my grandmother's face was calm, her breathing unlabored. But underneath the closed lids, her eyeballs fidgeted as though they were tracking a hummingbird buzzing from flower to flower.

My mother sat on the edge of the bed and picked up her mother's rope-veined hands.

"Your *Ama* was just at the hospital," she said, gently caressing the papery skin riddled with the needlemarks of intravenous lines and purplish bruises of blood draws.

I stood there in my shorts and T-shirt, flip-flops firmly planted on the plush carpet. The last time I had seen my *Ama*—"Grandmother" in Chinese—was a year earlier; she was in her kitchen, cooking up a storm of her signature dishes *afritada*, *mechado*, *arroz caldo*, and *empanada*. She was a short woman with thick gray hair held in a tight bun, large, obsidian eyes, and naturally tanned skin. For as long as I had known her, she had been a ball of perpetual energy, her pear-shaped body bouncing around her house the entire day, cooking, cleaning, chatting on the phone, playing mahjong like there was no tomorrow. I found it difficult to reconcile this with the shriveled old woman underneath the sheets, the emaciated impostor claiming to be my *Ama*, the loose skin under her chin quivering like a deflated balloon with each breath.

"Well, son," my mother said, eyeing me. "Aren't you going to examine her?"

I didn't want to be there, and I knew it showed in the way I crossed my hands over my chest and stood closer to the door than the bed.

"But Ma, I don't have my stethoscope . . . my equipment."

My mother pursed her lips tightly and turned her attention back to Celedonia.

Realizing that my mother wasn't about to let me leave, I inched closer and sat on the other side of the bed. I reached out a tentative hand and touched my grandmother's shoulder.

"*Ama*," I said softly. "It's me . . . I'm back."

She did not react so I shook her gently, leaned closer, and whispered in her ear to make sure that she heard me. The flickering movement of her eyeballs slowed, but her lids remained shut.

"Your *Ama* has been unresponsive since she returned from the hospital," my mother said. "The doctor told us she just has a urinary tract infection and gave her some antibiotics. But something's not right . . . "

I took Celedonia's hand from my mother and felt the pulse on her wrist: weak, thready, too fast. My other hand absently felt for the penlight in the pocket of the white coat that was hanging in the closet of my apartment three thousand miles away.

"What do you need?" my mother asked.

I told her that I wanted to prop my grandmother's eyelid open to look at her pupils. My mother immediately got up from her perch and left the room, shutting the door gently behind her.

While I waited for her to return, I dug deep in my mind and tried to recall what Dr. Elise Coletta had told me a few months earlier. Elise, as she liked to be called by her students, was the amiable physician I shadowed for a couple of afternoons during the required geriatric medicine rotation. As the geriatric specialist of the faculty, she was tasked to teach residents and medical students how to evaluate and treat elderly patients. Before I met with Elise, interns who had already gone through the experience spoke of dark, depressing nursing homes with carpets riddled with mysterious stains, stale air thick with the smell of urine, and decrepit old people tugging at their white coats as though they held their salvation. But when I got there, I found that it wasn't as bad as I had expected. For sure the place wasn't cheery, but while I trailed Elise as she went from room to room discussing a litany of medical problems in the elderly, little old ladies wearing lipstick and rouge looked up and smiled at me from their wheelchairs and walkers. We walked past rooms decked with pictures of grand-children and great-grandchildren, and in the activity room a group of seniors clapped and sang along while a man in suspenders played "You Are My Sunshine" on the banjo. As a young resident, I found it all rather strange, and the medical conditions Elise seemed most passionate about—dementia, delirium, pressure ulcers, and end-of-life care—vaguely interesting though decidedly unchallenging, unappeal-ing, and, well, unsexy. So I trudged behind her, listening with half my mind as the other half kept track of when I'd be able to leave, go home, and prepare for my cardiology rotation.

Back in Arcadia, alone with my *Ama*, not knowing how to help her, I wished I had paid better attention to Elise, asked more questions, taken more notes. But instead of Elise's pearls of wisdom, what came to mind was the way smug residents like me treated patients like my grand-mother. In the university hospital where I trained (and most other teach-ing hospitals for that matter), Celedonia was what we called a GOMER (get out of my ER), medical slang for an elderly patient perceived to be a waste of space in the emergency room. More often than not, we would roll our eyes at the sight of a GOMER being pulled out of an ambulance, strapped to a gurney, confused as a cow on Astroturf. They were the patients nobody wanted, the ones internists tried to turf to surgeons, surgeons tried to turf to neurologists, and neurologists tried to turf back to the internists. I would have tried that trick if I had anyone more com-petent to turf my grandmother to, but it was only us in that room.

It has been said that there is no point in a physician's career when he or she is surer of himself or herself than the period between the end of internship and the first humbling incident—an unexpected death or a punctured lung from a misplaced needle—that forces the cocky young physician to come face-to-face with his or her ignorance. I hadn't expected the humiliation to happen to me so soon, and cer-tainly not with my own grandmother.

My mother returned with a large flashlight that looked more suited to flood a dark campground than for peering into an old woman's eyes. Still, I took it from her and tested the reaction of Celedonia's pupils, which turned out to be just fine. But as I was about to shut off the light, I noticed a strange tinge on her eye's sclera, the white area around the iris. I asked my mother to draw the curtain open to let more daylight in. Like turning on a lamp, my grandmother's sclera glowed bright yellow.

I reached out my hand and rested it on Celedonia's abdomen while I kept my eyes trained to her face. I gently applied pressure over her belly button: no reaction. As I had been taught in medical school, I mentally dissected her abdomen into four quadrants and systematically palpated each section, picturing the organs that resided underneath the thin layers of skin and muscles. When I moved my hand over the right upper quadrant, the flickering movements of her eyeballs returned, followed by the slightest of winces. I pressed harder and to my surprise, her hand suddenly rose and spanked the back of my hand as though I had done something naughty.

I glanced at my mother, who was staring at me; this was the first reaction she had seen Celedonia make since she fell ill.

"What did you do?" she said incredulously. "I mean, how did you make her do that?"

"I'm not sure," I said, shaking my head thoughtfully like my medical school professors used to do during rounds. "But I think there's something wrong with her liver . . . or gallbladder. Did she get an ultrasound at the hospital?"

When I returned to Providence, I sifted through the binder that Elise had given me and read an article about the demography of the aging U.S. population. In 2011, the first baby boomers will turn 65. Unlike

my grandmother, who was a child of the Depression and had nine children, the boomers are better educated and wealthier but have fewer
children to depend on. As I read on, what struck me the most was
their sheer number: in the next twenty-five years as all boomers reach
retirement age, the number of Americans sixty-five years and older
will surge from 37 million to over 70 million.

According to the Institute of Medicine, while older adults currently constitute only 12 percent of the U.S. population, they account
for a whopping 26 percent of all physician visits, 35 percent of all hospital stays, 34 percent of all prescriptions, and 38 percent of all emergency medical service responses. In 2030, the elderly will constitute
20 percent of the U.S. population and this onslaught could bring our
health care system to its knees. Geriatricians are physicians who spe-
cialize in the care of the complex problems of elderly patients like my
grandmother. In 2007, there were just over 7,100 physicians certified in
geriatric medicine to care for the 37 million older Americans. By 2030,
it is estimated that there will be a need for 36,000 geriatricians. If the
laws of supply and demand were at work, one would assume that medical students should be training in droves to become geriatric medicine
practitioners, but not so.

I can still clearly recall the baffled look on my residency program
director's face when I told him I was considering geriatric medicine as
a career. I had already told my co-residents and friends about my interest, and their nearly universal reaction was, "Why?" Before I verbalized
my intention to anyone, I had asked myself the same question. When
internists choose to enter a fellowship in, say, cardiology or oncology,
they invest an additional two or three years of their post-residency
life to become specialists, and in return, they reap the rewards of this
investment in the form of higher status, better incomes, and other
perks. Geriatrics is the only specialty that actually causes a *decrease* in
physician income with additional training. This paradoxical relation-

ship between geriatric training and income is explained by the fact that older patients are time-consuming to care for and tend to have more complex medical problems. Coupled with this, reimbursements from Medicare and Medicaid, the largest payers of health care for elderly Americans, remain low and are in danger of further cuts, thus perpetuating the marginalization of geriatric medicine as a specialty. This is in sharp contrast to the system in Britain, where physician compensation scales up with the age of the patient. Not surprisingly, geriatrics is the most popular specialty among British medical students.

If not me, then *who* will care for the deluge of older American patients like Celedonia? If none of the bright, idealistic students in my class choose the road less traveled over the ROAD paved in gold, what will happen to our parents, grandparents, and the rest of the baby boomers? Some policymakers say that until the incomes of geriatricians are adjusted to approach those of cardiologists, gastroenterologists, and other specialists, fewer and fewer young physicians will enter the field and the shortage will worsen. Others say that more than the income discrepancy, our society's denial of aging and aversion to the old keeps the best and brightest young minds from becoming geriatricians. Still others say that the problem is more basic: the practice of geriatrics is like trying to put out fires that have been smoldering for years and will not die—chronic diseases like dementia, arthritis, and osteoporosis cannot be cured—making it inherently less satisfying to the physician who signed up for the healing, not the firefighting, profession. Young doctors want to heal and to cure, not to be mere stewards of the incurable—doctors of none.

To cure sometimes, to relieve often, and to comfort always was the aphorism of Edward Trudeau, an American physician who fought the then-incurable white plague: tuberculosis. Like others, I too originally wanted to become a healer. But Elise and Celedonia taught me that when a cure is not possible, to relieve pain and to provide comfort in times of suffering are equally worthy goals. Now that we have all but conquered tuberculosis through public health interventions and potent antibiotics, I wonder whether we will ever vanquish the seemingly incurable medical and social ills that come with aging, and resolve the even more daunting issue of who will care for our nation's elderly.

I saw Elise at a geriatrics conference near the end of my fellowship training. I recalled the surprised smile on her face when I thanked her for inspiring me to go into geriatrics. That was the last time I saw her. About a year later, Dr. Coletta died after a brief illness at the age of forty-seven, too young for anyone but especially for someone who had devoted her career to the care of the elderly and her life to inspiring young physicians like me to share her passion.

Celedonia was found to have terminal hepatic cancer. Her nine children looked back at the full life she had led and decided to ensure her comfort as she made the transition from that life to a dignified death. According to a German proverb, death is the poor man's doctor. But when death came for Celedonia and found her surrounded by the people who loved her, she was a very rich woman indeed.

GOOD INTENTIONS

Sandeep Jauhar

James Irey hailed from Trinidad, and though he had spent much of his adult life in the United States, he retained a calm, elegant island air—quiet and dignified, like a Rastafarian. When I first met him in the emergency room at Columbia Presbyterian Medical Center in Manhattan, where he had been admitted with congestive heart failure due to sarcoidosis, a chronic disease that had infiltrated his heart and lungs, it was immediately obvious he was near the end of his life. In his late fifties, bony thin, with salt-and-pepper braids, he was lying on a gurney in an almost meditative pose, as if his focusing on his labored breathing were crowding out all distractions. A combined heart-lung transplant was probably his only hope to live longer than a few months, but when I brought it up, he refused to consider it. He said he would rather die than undergo such an invasive treatment.

After reviewing the case with my colleagues, I told Irey that he needed a cardiac catheterization, in which a thin, flexible tube is threaded through a vein in the groin and into the right side of the heart to measure the pressures inside the heart and lungs. Data from the catheterization would help us treat Irey medically, but just as important—though I didn't tell him this—the data would help us determine whether Irey was eligible for a transplant. If the pressures were too high, then for technical reasons a transplant would not be feasible. What was the harm, I thought, in getting more information? Why not just do the evaluation and deal with his objections later?

With prodding from his wife, Irey reluctantly agreed, and he underwent the procedure the following day. In the early evening, I reviewed the results with Santo Russo, a young Italian cardiologist I had been working with. Though Russo had completed his fellowship only a few years earlier, with his gentle manner and good, European common sense—pragmatic, direct, rational—he was someone I looked up to and aspired to emulate. Poring over the catheterization report, Russo pointed out a critical discrepancy in the measurements. The pressure in Irey's lungs was high, but whether the elevation was reversible or not—a crucial factor in deciding whether Irey was a transplant candidate—was open to interpretation. To settle the issue, Russo said, the procedure would have to be repeated. Initially, I demurred, wondering whether it was worth doing given Irey's opposition to a transplant, but Russo insisted we try to convince Irey, for his own sake.

A patient's right to self-determination is the cornerstone of medical ethics, but as any experienced doctor will tell you, it has its complications. As a doctor, when do you let your patient make a bad decision? How hard should you push him to change his mind? What if it is a matter of life and death? Are you obligated to try to save him from himself? At the same time, who are you to tell him what is right or wrong? Isn't your patient better equipped to make that judgment?

Russo and I went to talk to Irey. He was in bed, wearing bright red

pajamas, a stark contrast to the air of grim expectation that perme-
ated the room. Thin plastic tubing delivering supplemental oxygen
pressed tightly against his sunken cheeks, ending in tiny prongs jut-
ting into flaring brown nostrils. His wife was with him, sitting quietly;
she barely acknowledged us when we entered. Russo greeted Irey and
asked him how he was feeling. Irey said that he was still uncomfortable, especially in the right upper quadrant of the abdomen (where
fluid was probably backing up in his liver due to heart failure), and that
he was so exhausted he could hardly move. He said it without self-pity,
though it was a self-pitying remark. He inquired about the results of
the catheterization. Russo matter-of-factly told him that the measurements were inconclusive and would have to be repeated.

Irey closed his eyes. "I can't go through that again," he rasped
softly. "It takes too much out of me. Just treat me with medicines."

"Yes, well, we are going to do that," Russo replied with a slight
accent. "But if you require a transplant, then we will need that information."

"No transplant," Irey said, shaking his head wearily. He said it
with even more conviction than he had the previous evening. He
asked how long he could live without one.

"You are very sick," Russo said gravely. "I cannot really say, but
your lifespan will be limited."

"How limited?" Irey said. He seemed prepared to hear even the
worst prognosis.

"The most severe problem is with your lungs," Russo said. "We are
not lung experts. You really should ask the pulmonologists."

"I'm asking for your opinion. How long do I have?"

Russo shrugged. "Maybe a year," he said.

Irey didn't miss a beat. "That's fine, I'll take it. No transplant. And
so I won't have to have the procedure tomorrow?"

Russo shot me a glance conveying he understood that convincing Irey would be more difficult than he originally imagined. Leaning against a bedside table, where Russo's dinner tray was sitting untouched, he said, "Well, probably not. If you say 'no transplant,' then it puts a different light on this hospitalization."

"Then I can go home?"

"May I ask why you don't want a transplant?"

"I don't want to go through that," Irey said, waving his hand to dismiss the suggestion. "I don't want no one cutting me open."

"Your lungs are scarred. There is a lot of fibrosis—" Russo began.

"But you will still treat me?" Irey interrupted.

"But this is not what I would call treatment," Russo replied firmly. "It is more, if you can understand what I mean, palliation." The look in Irey's eyes told me that he understood. "It is like giving Tylenol for a fever. You give the Tylenol and the fever goes away, but you are not better."

"But you will still treat me?" Irey pressed. "If I say no, you'll still give me treatment to help me live as long as possible."

"Well, yes, of course," Russo said with a trace of exasperation, as if it were an absurd question. "But there is treatment at the medical level and treatment at the transplant level. There is only so much we can do without a transplant. When you crash an engine, sometimes you can fix it, but sometimes the whole thing has to be replaced. This is the situation that you are now in. If it was just your heart, we could treat it. It is not a good situation, but we can handle it. But your lungs are the more serious problem. That you will have to discuss with the lung specialists. They will talk to you tomorrow. I hope you will have a similar conversation with them as we are having today."

"But you say one year," Irey said hopefully.

"I don't know," Russo replied quickly. "It could be less. You must ask the lung doctors. I don't want you to say, 'Dr. Russo told me I have one year to live.' Let us just say, a few months to one year."

"I understand," Irey said, settling back, looking a bit more relaxed. "I won't tell anyone."

Mrs. Irey had a world-weary look, as if she had heard this discussion many times before. "Our understanding was that he could be put on a transplant list, and then we could decide," she said. Russo shook his head. "It does not work that way," he said. "We need a firm commitment from the patient before we can put him on the list."

"But how can he commit when he doesn't know what it means medically?" Mrs. Irey asked. I glanced at Irey, who appeared spent and preoccupied once again with his breathing.

"That is fine, but he has to buy into the concept. Even then, there is a low chance he will be accepted. For technical reasons we may not be able to—"

"Please forgive me for being so blunt," Mrs. Irey interrupted, "but in your opinion, would it be worth the expense, the effort? Will he be better off?" Irey looked away, as if he had heard this line of inquiry before.

"I think so," Russo said carefully. "I can only speak about heart transplant because that is what I do, where the successes are great. People do very well. I mean, for the first six months there is a lot of intensive monitoring, and he has to take a lot of medicine for a very long time, some for life—"

"But will he be better off?" Mrs. Irey demanded again. "Will he have less suffering than if he says no right now?"

"There is an acute phase and a chronic phase," Russo began. "For six months, it is a critical period. For the first couple of weeks he may even do worse. Obviously, they have to cut him open. But the end result can be very good."

I shifted uncomfortably. Russo, it seemed to me, was painting a much rosier picture of organ transplantation than was warranted.

"I don't think he understands what it means," Mrs. Irey said, as her husband continued to stare meditatively at the wall. "I'm not sure he can make a decision with the information that he has."

Of course, this came as no surprise. Hospitalized patients have a hard time properly weighing their options under the best of circumstances. In a situation like this, where the stakes were so high and Irey so ill, how could we expect him to make such a difficult choice?

After a few more minutes, the issue still unresolved, Russo left. I stayed behind to remove the dressing on Irey's groin, where the catheter had been inserted. Irey groaned as the adhesive pulled on the trapped hairs. Slowly, methodically, I worked off the clear bandage, unwilling to give it a quick tug to end the pain.

"I know this is probably unfair, and I'm sorry to put you in this difficult position, but what would you do?" Mrs. Irey asked me.

This question had been posed to me many times before during my medical training. As I had learned, sometimes patients and their families want to hear their options and make their own decisions, but sometimes they just want doctors to tell them what to do. Of course, I realized Irey wasn't the one asking for my advice, but there was enough uncertainty in the room to convince me that coming down strongly in favor of a transplant might persuade Irey into making what I still thought was the right choice.

"I think you should have the catheterization and try to get on the transplant list," I said, looking straight at Irey. "Frankly, the chances that you will be offered a transplant are pretty slim. If the answer is no, at least you know you exhausted all the options. Who knows, six months from now, you might have second thoughts. Then you might be sicker and it will be harder to start the process all over again. Besides, it's just another catheterization—"

"Have you had it?" Irey whispered.

"It's a routine test," I said.

"Have you had it?" he said again.

"No, I can't say I have," I replied.

"Then you can't tell me what it's like, right?"

"Fair enough," I said. Any risk or discomfort was his to bear, not mine.

Once he had extracted this admission from me, Irey's countenance softened. "I'll think about it overnight," he said. "Will you come talk with me in the morning?" I said I would. "I would like that very much," he said.

At home that night, I found myself worrying about the advice I had given. Nothing about Irey's case suggested that he'd get the survival benefit that Russo had promised. How many patients like Irey, debilitated and weak, terminally ill with sarcoidosis, had been studied in transplant trials? Not many, I was willing to bet. In advising Irey to pursue a transplant, we were operating in the realm of intuition and faith. And, of course, so was Irey. We were pitting our faith against his.

Late the following morning I was walking through the cardiac care unit when I caught a glimpse of a patient with salt-and-pepper braids. He was on a ventilator, in a tangle of wires and tubes. Alarmed, I pulled a resident aside, who told me that Irey had just been brought in from the catheterization lab. A balloon-tipped catheter inflated during the procedure had apparently punctured his pulmonary artery, causing his blood pressure to drop precipitously. He had started coughing up blood, and then had had a cardiac arrest on the operating table. I grabbed the chart, looking for a procedure note (there was none). I paged Russo but he did not call me back.

Then I saw Mrs. Irey. She came in, carrying a bag. I went over to her and grasped her hand, trying to think of something appropriate to say, but it escaped me. "He decided to have the procedure after you left," she said, grief-stricken. "We didn't see you this morning, so we told the other doctors."

My thoughts were like leaves fluttering in the wake of a speeding car. For the remainder of the day, I tried to concentrate on my other patients, but the admonishments kept flooding in, even as I tried to resist them. *Why did you convince Irey against his better judgment? Aren't you responsible for what happened?*

Irey pulled on for a couple of days, but his condition eventually spiraled downward and he died. Mrs. Irey never mentioned the conversation Russo and I had had with her husband, one that undoubtedly led to his premature death, other than to say, "He never wanted a transplant. Maybe he knew better than us."

And perhaps he did. It sometimes still amazes me, more than a decade into my medical career, how much power doctors have to affect patients' lives, for better or for worse. With that power comes a tremendous responsibility to wield it wisely, sparingly, with humility. Every patient teaches a lesson, and the lesson James Irey taught me was that a doctor's words can have terrible consequences. A doctor's advice means a lot, and like most patients, Irey in the end was unable to reject it. Though our intentions were good, the outcome to which Russo and I undoubtedly contributed was horrible. But tragedy is a powerful lesson. Doctors often think we know better than our patients, but of course, this isn't always true.

EN ROUTE

Abigail Zuger

*I*t is a balmy July night in New York City, 1981. The fluorescent lights in the hallway of ward 16E of Bellevue Hospital never dim, but after dinner things slowly settle down. Visitors leave at eight. The nurses change shift at eleven. By midnight, everything is quiet. An intern balancing blood tubes, needles, and syringes on a clipboard heads into a darkened room. The night nurse wheels the medication cart down to the far end of the ward and begins to give out the night meds.

In a four-bed room way at the far end of the hall, a young woman named Nilda is standing next to her bed looking out the window.

She knows the view well: river, tugboats, and bridge to the left, sunrise over Brooklyn to the right, moonrise over Queens straight ahead. She has been in this room for three weeks now. Two months ago she spent two weeks over on 16W and got to see the sun set beside the Empire State

Building. A month before that, it was 16E again, but only for a few days. She had to leave early that time, to go pay her rent.

Her problem never changes. It is fever, always fever. No one can figure out why. She knows the routine now as well as the interns do, and she knows pretty much all the interns now, too. She meets them in rotation night after night, when her fever spikes high and they come in to draw her blood. But the tests for all the various problems heroin addicts can get—endocarditis, hepatitis, cellulitis, pneumonia, blood clots—just keep coming back negative. So, after a few weeks in the hospital she gathers her things together, feeling a little stronger from the regular meals and the bed rest and the forced detox, and goes back home. Back to her apartment, that dump. Back to heroin. Back to fevers, sweats, feeling weak. Then back to Bellevue. This has become her routine. It's not so bad. Sometimes she helps the nurses feed the other patients in her room—three old, old ladies, one Spanish, one black, one Chinese, all asleep, all snoring.

Nilda is waiting for the intern. She was 103.8 at the last temperature check. They always draw blood for culture when she is this hot. That's how they check for endocarditis, an infection in the heart from shooting drugs. By now she must have had blood cultures a hundred times, and they are always negative. They all know she doesn't have endocarditis. But still they draw more blood, the nice ones probing for the few good veins she has left in her hands and arms, the impatient ones just going for the big veins in her groin or her neck. Jerks. But she always lets them. She has no choice. She knows she is sick. She is getting scared. She used to be a big woman, even with the drugs. Now she is a stick. Her old man moved out last month. The city took the kids long ago. She might as well be here as anywhere.

The overhead light in the room snaps on. The old ladies keep snoring.

"Hi," says the intern. Both of them blink in the sudden light. "It's only me."

And indeed, it was only me, three weeks into my internship, midway through a long, sleepless night on call. I was up all night, every third night, those days, zooming around the corridors of Bellevue fueled exclusively by nerves and fear. You couldn't even get a cup of coffee in that place from the time the cafeteria closed at 7 p.m. till 3 a.m., when a truck that peddled snacks pulled into the back parking lot. I had drawn blood from poor Nilda so many times by then that I could navigate her skinny hands and wrists without even looking. Among us all, we had drawn at least forty sets of blood cultures, all negative, and yet my resident made us draw more. We all knew that he had pretty much no idea what to do with Nilda, but he had to do something, of course, and so we kept drawing her blood.

This was now more than twenty-five years ago. In theory, I had been a doctor for about seven weeks. In actuality, I still had quite some time to go. In actuality, I'm still working on it. Sitting at my clinic desk in the mornings, looking at my list of patients for the day, I catch myself thinking, "Good lord, these people need a doctor." Instead, what they have is me, an amphibious creature still in the process of evolving. Sometimes what I am at the moment is exactly what a patient needs. Sometimes the need and the reality are so wildly disparate that catastrophe results. And sometimes, as years pass, we grow into each other, water against stone, a long, slow process.

I don't know that I am particularly backward in my evolutionary progress. I suspect I am right in the middle of the pack. There are some practitioners—you may well have met one or two yourself—who never make it at all. Forget the diploma on the wall: medical school comes and goes far too quickly to have much of an impact. Almost everyone is aware of this fact but medical students, who take themselves and their perceived mission (to memorize every piece of information they will ever have to know) very seriously. In my day we loaded ourselves up with notebooks and index cards; now they use portable computers. Either way, students hoard facts and treatment guidelines like squirrels hoard nuts, hiding them in accessible places against the coming of that long, dark winter between graduation and retirement, during which they assume they will never be able to be uncertain or to ask anyone a question ever again.

Little do they know, poor things, that medical facts have a shelf life just like nuts. Most of them will spoil before they are ever used. New ones will show up unannounced. A study some years ago methodically evaluated the lifespan of a body of medical knowledge and found a half-life of forty-five years. In other words, half of what you learn in medical school is obsolete by the time you are in your sixties (and presumably think you know what you are doing). Nobody is going to tell you which half.

My particular circumstances are even more extreme: I spend my workdays taking care of patients with a disease that did not exist when I was in school. Nothing like AIDS had ever been dreamed of. I graduated and landed in an entirely new world, full of naked, unprocessed facts without journals or textbooks to organize them for us. Nilda baffled us, and so did the dozens and then hundreds of patients who came after her, clogging the system with their dire illnesses and our inability to figure them out. Patients came to the hospital and stayed for weeks and months; if we sent them home, they came right back. The disease had no name back then, let alone any algorithms for thinking its problems through. It stripped doctors of everything that medical school tried to teach them: their facts and their confidence simultaneously. It changed everything.

Sometimes I amuse myself thinking back to two of the attending doctors I met during medical school, who epitomized fairly standard operating modes. Call them Dr. Data and Dr. Confidence. Neither would last a moment in my world.

Dr. Data was a fact man: he had maintained the mind-set of a medical student from graduation onward. He was evidence-based all the way: he practiced as the very latest studies and nomograms told him to. He aimed to provide the best care to all comers, by which he generally meant the same care, validated in large clinical trials, based on scientific evidence.

Dr. Data was a cardiologist. Lean, trim, a runner, he refused to take care of anyone who smoked. He was quite proud of himself for this unusual detail of his practice; he had thought of it all by himself. Sitting in his pleasant consultation room, he would break the news to would-be patients with a certain straight-faced glee. I could have sworn he sent the occasional wink toward the student observing from a corner.

"First things first," he would tell the patient after the initial history and physical exam. "If you smoke, you are just wasting my time. We are just wasting each other's time. Go home, quit smoking, make an appointment to come back. I can't do anything for you if you undo it all with cigarettes. Good to see you." He would stand, shake hands, open the door, and the patient would head out to the great beyond without a peep. I don't know how many of them came back. Should Dr. Data still be in practice, under Medicare's current plans to pay physicians for getting good results and penalize them for getting bad ones he would be in clover.

Were he to be sitting in my chair on a Monday morning, banishing patients from his presence for their array of addictions, bad habits, and human frailties, he would be out of work by Tuesday noon.

Dr. Confidence operated at the opposite end of the spectrum. He made his progress through the hospital abdomen first, bow tie second, starched white coat buttoned from top to bottom, sleeves secured with cufflinks around pudgy wrists. He seemed to know no actual medicine at all. On rounds with Dr. Confidence the usual patterns were reversed: we students were the ones who taught him a thing or two, quoting the newest studies as he nodded appreciatively and made notes on file cards. Not that he ever used the information: his patients kept getting antique tests, old drugs given in weird ways the other attendings had abandoned long ago. Dr. Confidence was a standing joke. We pitied his patients.

Imagine my surprise when an idle conversation at a high school reunion unearthed the incredible fact that one of my friends—sharp, sophisticated, nobody's fool—was one of them. That she had actually sought him out, on the strong recommendation of her aunt, whose life Dr. Confidence had saved. The aunt had been deathly ill with a disease called (here my friend, an English major and science hater, stuttered a little but pressed on) systemic lupus erythematosus. Dr. Confidence had saved her life by treating her with a powerful new drug, prednisone. The whole family saw him now. He was great. They worshipped him.

I just stared at her. Prednisone for lupus. A fourth-grader with a copy of the *Merck* manual would know to give someone prednisone for lupus. That was the drug you gave, and it wasn't new, not by a long shot, not by decades. But Dr. Confidence in all his starched self-assured godlike presence had managed to transform a completely straightforward clinical transaction into an act of personal triumph.

I enjoy the image of Dr. Confidence sitting at my desk, white-coated, bow-tied, trying to preserve the illusion of divine omniscience and control with a patient who was diagnosed with AIDS twenty years ago, who was told then that he had eighteen months to live, and who has in the interim made his own survival his life's career. Our patients have no time or tolerance for medical bloviation. They are simply not in the mood. They have watched the sands shift so wildly, they have defied so many dire, confident predictions, that the only certain way to gain their confidence is to share their uncertainties.

But if neither Dr. Data nor Dr. Confidence would survive in my world, then who does? If a doctor is not to be a scientist or a shaman, what then?

I am certainly not the first to ask this question. One widely quoted answer was voiced by Dr. Francis W. Peabody, an eminent Boston physician who told a class of Harvard students in 1925 that "the secret of the care of the patient is in caring for the patient." Nicely put, but still, what exactly does that mean? Who is the doctor to be, in this caring role? A parent, a friend, a policeman? A guardian angel, an alter ego, a parole officer? There are no prototypes that fit completely, and no rules for creating new ones. There is only trial and error.

My biggest success to date, I think, has been with Audrey, long a supremely difficult patient. She is a small, flamboyant woman, with a gigantic wardrobe of wigs, scarves, dresses, boots, and snakeskin pants. She dresses according to mood, some days as prim and demure as any youngish senior citizen (her records say she is sixty-three, she admits to sixty-seven, but sometimes forgets and gives dates that calculate out to sixty-nine). Other days she is a teenager, and others a movie star. In fact, Audrey started out life as a man, but no one has to know that piece of information. She refuses to discuss it.

Whoever she is on any particular day, Audrey stays in control; that goes for her own behavior, and for everyone else's, too. She takes her AIDS medications precisely, and her infection has been under optimal control for years. She watches her weight. She has a slew of therapists, whom she sees on an as-needed basis. Her cocaine use is episodic—pretty much alternating with her stints in therapy. She does not like to be confined by arbitrary, man-made barriers such as, say, appointment times, and pretty much shows up in my office whenever she feels the need.

There was a time when I would see her name on my list and groan at the prospect of another mentally bruising session with Audrey and her achy knee, her recurrent headaches, her weight loss, her weight gain, her troubled relationships, her difficulty urinating—and no, no examination of her private parts is ever permitted. Audrey was impossible. She knew exactly what she needed, be it antibiotics or nutritional supplements, or migraine medication, or the latest prescription diet drug, or an X-ray of her perfectly normal knee, and battered me till I finally said yes, just to cut my losses and get on to the next patient.

One month a few years ago it all got out of hand. Audrey was in the clinic every day, sometimes twice a day, for every passing twinge. She was anxious, she finally confided. She had a big show coming up. She was in a cabaret class and the final exam was to be a public performance.

It was our clinic nurse who had the great idea. And so, one evening a few weeks later the nurse, the clinic manager, and I forked over a cover charge, ordered our two-drink minimum in a little dark cellar nightclub, and watched Audrey slink up on stage in a sequined gown and croon "Smoke Gets in Your Eyes." She was truly wonderful. She was triumphant. She brought down the house, and we gave her a standing ovation.

From that night on, Audrey has been a changed person with us. She has stopped banging on doors and waits patiently to be seen. She makes and keeps appointments. She tells me she is blessed to have me in her life. She has actually said the following words: "Anything you say, Doctor." Suddenly she is happy to behave like a patient and let me behave like a doctor, all because I once treated her like a person, not a patient. Is that, perhaps, the secret of caring for the patient?

Or is it even simpler than that? Way back in that long-ago July of my internship year, Nilda and I spent an awful lot of time together, for the simple reason that my blood-drawing skills were not, at that point, all they might have been. I knew Nilda's hands and wrists up and down, but I still had terrible trouble getting her blood. Those were the days when I actually dreamed about drawing her blood, I dreaded it so much: I dreaded the pain I inflicted, and the bruises I produced, and the occasional humiliating outcome of having to confess the next morning that I had simply been unable to get it. I never went for the big veins in the groin or neck like some of the others did because I was far too scared. Instead, I wrapped hot towels around Nilda's poor thin hands and hoped the veins would appear.

One early morning, waiting in Nilda's room for her towel-encased hands to yield a usable vein, I noticed that her covered dinner tray was still lying on the bedside table, untouched. "I hate fish," she said, shrugging. As it happens, I hate fish too. I looked at my watch. It was 3 a.m., just the hour for the life-saving snack truck to be pulling up to the hospital's back door. I was beyond starving. I never ate meals, back then. There was never time.

I ran down to the truck and bought two giant doughnuts and two cups of coffee. We ate and drank side by side, sitting on the edge of Nilda's bed.

That Christmas I got a card from Nilda, addressed to me at the hospital. Shortly thereafter came a phone call from the emergency room of some hospital in Brooklyn, where she had shown up, suddenly blind in one eye. She had told them I was her doctor. After that I never heard from or about her again.

Not infrequently, these days, when I hear my colleagues spinning fulsome phrases about the doctor-patient relationship, or when I think about all the forces that can help a poor frightened intern crawl a few yards out of the primal muck of confusion onto a firmer shore, I wonder if anyone else realizes that sometimes it can all boil down to a doughnut.

A FIRE, DELIBERATELY SET

Peggy Sarjeant

It is the Saturday before Easter and exactly ten years since my friend Karen was buried. Her body lies in a tiny cemetery outside of Buffalo Gap, Texas, beneath a red bud tree that, if it has been a warm spring, is by now in delicate bloom. The purple irises that grow wild over the graves are likely also blooming, as are the paintbrush, like clusters of orange flame in the new grass.

On this same day, twenty years ago, I attended another funeral. Mandi had been my first patient to die. Though I had seen death in medical school—stab wounds, gunshot wounds, a hatchet wedged into a heart—I always felt three steps removed. Not because of the violent methods by which the people died but, rather, simply because they were patients. In medical school I had been taught I must set myself apart. I had been conditioned for separation.

Eight months into my residency, Mandi changed everything. She was responsible for the challenge to my carefully constructed professional guard. She, a patient—and a teenager, no less—wormed her way into my heart.

I don't know where Mandi is buried, but at this time of year I always wonder. I'd like to visit. I'd like to tell her I'm not a doctor anymore and that, all these years later, she is the reason. I'd like to tell her about Karen. And I'd like her to know I am grateful.

At first, I hated Adolescent Medicine. Teenagers unnerved me. They were rude and condescending; hormones raced through their brains like acid through plastic, and left them menacing and sullen. One minute they were detached and the next so close you could smell their insecurity. Every one of them stood at the edge of some catastrophic arousal I'd worked my whole life to avoid. In 1988, I was twenty-seven and an intern at Children's Hospital, in Seattle. I had chosen to study Pediatrics because adult illnesses were too often the result of self-destructive behavior and because sick adults were, well, whiney. And even though Pediatrics included Adolescent Medicine, as for teenagers, I planned to ban anyone with pubic hair from my future practice. I preferred babies—sick infants with IVs sticking up from their scalps. I preferred patients who didn't talk.

But residency training didn't accommodate my discrimination. Late one Friday afternoon, I admitted Mandi. She was fourteen years old. Her doctor said she had mono and sent her to the hospital for fluids and pain control. He was certain she would be home in twenty-four hours.

Mandi's neck bulged with lymph nodes as big as golf balls; when I looked in her throat, I saw nothing but bulging pink tonsils networked with purple veins. I hooked up the saline and the morphine. Mandi sat on the edge of her bed and spit her saliva into a yellow-striped dishcloth because her throat was so sore she couldn't swallow.

Mandi didn't go home. By Monday morning, a cauliflowerlike growth hung down in front of her tonsils. A smaller version of the same thing could be seen in one of her nostrils. By Wednesday, the nasal mass protruded and lay gleaming against her upper lip. Specialists clustered like flies around Mandi's chart. More tests were ordered. Whatever she had was growing fast and no one—not the ENT docs, pulmonologists, gastroenterologists, or the oncologists—understood what was happening. But everyone knew Mandi didn't have mono.

Mandi called her brother and asked him to gather her homework. That first week she read *The Catcher in the Rye* and *The Heart Is a Lonely Hunter*. While the tumors grew down her throat and out her nose, she worked on algebra and wrote a whole essay for World History. Mandi talked to her parents and to her brother. Her friends and teachers made hospital visits and she talked to them, too. She even tried to talk to me.

At first, given my biases, I left her room as soon as I had gathered the information I needed. But as one week stretched into two, I lingered. With her hard work, her fortitude, and her engaging personality, Mandi began to unravel my preconceptions about teenagers. I had never met anyone so self-possessed, so uncomplaining, in the face of what was fast becoming a tragic medical nightmare. It was 5:30 p.m. on a Sunday and I was on call. I'd been in the hospital for thirty-six hours.

"Have you figured me out yet?" Mandi said.

"No. I'm sorry."

Her dinner—an anemic array of soft foods able to slip around the mass in her throat—sat before her, displayed in beige bowls.

She pushed the tray away. "Why did you decide to be a doctor?" she asked. "And don't tell me you wanted to help people."

I was exhausted. I sat on the edge of Mandi's bed. "It's true," I said. "I want to help people."

"Ha!" She poked a mound of vanilla pudding with a fork. "That's what they all say."

It occurred to me then that I'd never sat on a patient's bed. I'd never sat on a patient's bed because I had been taught that sitting on a patient's bed was unprofessional. In medical school—I had graduated only six months before—patient rounds had always been a stand-up affair: white coats and student doctors clutching 3 x 5 notecards; the attending physician standing in the doorway, his arms crossed over his chest. *An invasion of space*, we were told. *Suggests a familiarity that might be insulting. Implies an intimacy that is inappropriate.* Never mind that we were taught to poke every organ, to prod every private dark space; to ask questions that, in any other circumstance, would be considered the height of bad taste. No—as a physician, I should stand. Hold myself distant. Distance was necessary.

But there, in Mandi's room, I didn't move.

"Why did *you* want to be a doctor?" Mandi said.

I sighed. I'd always wanted to do something useful, something that mattered. I'm sure that desire was partly influenced by my parents' expectations for me to "succeed," but some of it was my own understanding. I had a deep desire to make a difference; I held to the ideal that I could change the world through selfless service. In college, I'd worked at a summer camp in Colorado that served disadvantaged Cajun kids from southern Louisiana and I seemed to have a unique ability to connect with others very different from myself. Decades later, medicine would lead me to East Africa and an adventure that is a whole separate story. Simply put, I believed God had given me gifts that I was expected to use. Helping others through medicine had somehow become the obvious choice.

"I was a good student and I liked science," I said. Mandi looked dubious. "I want to do something important, something personal." I shifted around on the brittle hospital sheets. "And I want to travel and live anywhere in the world I want to live," I said. "Being a doctor makes it all possible."

Doctors in training are warned not to grow too close to their patients for fear their professional judgment will end up tainted. We are told the human body is precious but that a physician's touch is best kept austere, limited to palpation and to percussion. We are taught that compassion is necessary, but must be delivered from a distance. All this, so that the decisions we make for our patients are not influenced by our own subjective—and, by suggestion, dangerous—emotions.

And so, when a physician speaks about her attachment to patients, about the very things that constitute compassion—commiseration, mercy, tenderness, and heart—she finds herself facing damning insinuations, dodging the vocabulary of mental illness. The terms "transference," "merging," and "codependence," in our current age of rampant pop psychology, have become household words. They describe specific, aberrant, and destructive psychological states. And certainly, they have no place in the professional doctor-patient relationship.

But, is there no room for the middle ground? For the interpretation that good care might include actions beyond the conscientious checking of a patient's lab results and the reporting of them at the bedside? That compassion might necessitate more than just lip service? That the expression of *agape*—that is, brotherly love—might actually benefit both patient and physician?

I had teachers that, in the same breath, as they warned us not to get too close, warned young physicians against the very real dangers of overactive defense mechanisms. Of the tendency to dehumanize, become callous; against the self-protection of indifference. The contradictions are enormous, and unavoidable.

How are doctors, who as human beings come face-to-face with others at their most vulnerable, to carry on? Do we compromise compassion in favor of professional convention? Do we turn our backs, substituting emotional bankruptcy for objectivity? Do we attempt to erase the contradictions with alcohol, or drugs; with a gun to our heads?

Perhaps, instead, we choose to abandon what we were taught. What we once embraced as students of the modern system.

Perhaps we return to the physician's roots. To a place of healing, rather than treatment. To a place of touch.

Perhaps we become human, instead of god.

Expressing love and compassion exacts a toll. We are not islands of objectivity. Distance and detachment, regardless of why they are cultivated, are defenses, not attributes. Attachment and emotional involvement are conscious choices—capable of fanning the flames of annihilation, or of regeneration.

"Burnout" has become a universally understood and uniquely professional cliché, yet the term originated in the language of firefighters. A "burnout" is defined as: "a fire, deliberately set inside a control line for the purpose of consuming fuel between the edge of a wildfire and the control line." In the context of medical practice, the consumed "fuel" stands for the physician; "wildfire," the patient; and "control line" the constraints of the current health care system.

What is not addressed is the phrase *a fire, deliberately set*. These words, in my construct, denote the purposeful departure from professional conventions. They lick around the edges of what might happen to a physician who consciously chooses to stray from expectations. They hint at the consumption—and, ironically, the renewal—that might occur should a physician choose a different path.

Karen and I met at Baylor University in the fall of 1981, as pledges to the Air Force ROTC–affiliated service organization, Angel Flight. Neither of us was the typical Baylor coed—Karen played soccer and rode horses, I had spent the last two summers in Colorado leading backpacking trips and teaching guitar—and we were both looking for a place to belong on a campus of plaid-clad Southern belles come to claim husbands.

Our respective applications revealed we had a lot in common. We both came from homes where expectations were high, where the burden of not disappointing our parents kept us fearful of failure and the appearance of weakness. I was the first from either side of my family to attend college; Karen was the youngest of three in a family where professional degrees were revered. Like me, Karen had been raised in the sprawling anonymity of suburban Dallas; like me, by the time she arrived at Baylor she had been smitten by the Far West and wanted, more than anything, to live in the mountains. But we were not yet ready to leave our home state and, not insignificantly, as Texas residents we received a substantial break on our tuition.

Karen and I took long rides over the prairie. Camped out in the hill country. Wandered a particular pecan grove gone wild. It was there, outside of Crawford, Texas, on a blustery November afternoon, that our friendship became firmly established. Pecans lay everywhere, all over the ground. We filled our jacket pockets, then our jeans pockets; we made pouches of the fronts of our sweatshirts and piled in pecans until we couldn't carry any more. I was comfortable in Karen's presence, and found an immense comfort in the fact I didn't have to explain myself. I can only assume Karen felt the same way.

"I love this time of day," Karen said. The setting sun had briefly appeared between a bank of clouds and the curve of the horizon.

"Me too," I said.

Everything stood out in Technicolor relief. The old orchard trees black and bare, like great gnarled fingers against the rose sky; the grass tawny and knee-high, the whole sea of it undulating like something alive and breathing beneath the wind. The colors more vivid in the low angle light; the deep scent of dirt, the rot of late autumn leaves. The sun, in its last winking moment, falling into oblivion.

"I call it a JOLF," Karen said, "how I feel at this time of day." I looked at her. "A Joy of Life Flash," she explained.

I smiled. I kicked at a chunk of limestone. I nodded. I understood, perfectly.

Those drives—sometimes evenings, sometimes mornings—became a weekend tradition. We often stopped at Little John's, a truck stop café outside of Waco that served the best hash browns in the world; other times we drove out to the lake, the scrub cedar and flinty hills to our back, and watched the sun sink into the prairie clouds. But always we spoke little, and asked for nothing more than the comfort of each other's company.

Karen and I exchanged Christmas cards and the occasional birthday greeting, but by 1994 we hadn't been in close contact until a mutual friend brought us back together again, for a fly-fishing trip. Karen and I had both been long married, and we each had two kids. Each of us had a daughter named Kristin. I was a pediatrician in Seattle; Karen, an environmental engineer in West Texas.

It was as if we had never parted. For a week, the three of us hiked among the glaciated peaks of the North Cascades; we cast our lines into crystalline pools. It rained, and rained, and rained, and all day, every day, we enjoyed the simple pleasure of companionship. At night, we holed up in a little cabin. We read. We shared photos. We cooked really good food and, now, six years after Mandi, we began to talk. About our kids, and how we thought they were marvels of intelligence, and gifted in all the areas we were not. About our professions and the challenges they posed. About our relationships, our homes; the dreams we'd fulfilled, and those we hadn't—yet. We laughed, and cried. We all felt we'd found the beginning of something new.

Despite the pleasure of being reunited, circumstances got in the way. Karen and I lived 2,500 miles apart and our busy lives as mothers, wives, and women with careers kept us from regular communication. That is, until July 1996, when I received a phone call. It was Karen; her voice small and distant, somehow higher-pitched and thin-edged. She told me of the tremendous headache that had plagued her for more than a month, of the diagnosis of migraines and her doctor's comment that this was a very common problem among "women your age." The treatments he had prescribed had not helped.

I learned, that night, that three months before, while mountain-biking with her husband in the hills not far from their home, Karen had had a seizure. A CT scan had been performed and was read as normal. A couple weeks later, at work, Karen had a second seizure. Now she was vomiting, and had pain that would wake her from sleep.

That first CT scan, in retrospect, showed a tiny tumor in Karen's right temporal lobe. But no one noticed it until the evening after she called me, when she had a third seizure—massive—in an emergency room parking lot. The subsequent biopsy revealed undifferentiated stage IV glioblastoma multiforme, the deadliest of brain tumors. Two to 5 percent of patients lived five years beyond diagnosis. Karen was thirty-four years old.

And so, I flew to Texas, knowing it was entirely possible that, once together, Karen and I might fall into our old pattern of shared silence. But Karen faced the loss of everything—of everyone—she loved. Silence, shared or otherwise, would not acknowledge the ugly and unendurable. It wouldn't address her fear that her faith in God was inadequate, that somehow she was responsible for her illness; it would only deny our friendship a last bloom of intimacy. And silence would betray everything I had learned from Mandi.

I started rounding a half hour earlier every morning so I had a few extra minutes for Mandi. Despite all my adolescent-related prejudices, I liked this kid. She was smart, and funny, and scathingly honest. She was not afraid to ask questions. She possessed a certain drivenness that I could respect, and that reminded me of myself at her age. Every time I walked into her room I felt something in my chest go soft, and hot. It was empathy; it was the fact that I could relate to her in a very personal way. Alas, against the warnings of my teachers, I had become attached.

I thought about Mandi on my commute home. I read everything I could find about small blue cell tumors, the nonspecific cell type—and the only, very nonspecific, diagnosis—a biopsy had revealed. I talked to the hospital pathologists, looked at her tissue samples under a microscope; I called a cancer specialist in Philadelphia and arranged for him to review her case. I wanted to do anything I could to help "figure her out"; I wanted her to get better. I wanted her to leave the hospital—not, as at first, to get her out of my hair, but to return to her family and friends. In the meantime, I looked forward to my nights on call. When my work was done, I sat on the edge of Mandi's bed and we talked.

One evening I found Mandi standing at the sink, looking into the mirror. She had been in the hospital three weeks. We were no closer to a useful diagnosis than the day she arrived.

"You look beautiful," I said. Mandi's long blond hair splayed out over her shoulders. Her flannel nightgown hung soft and rumpled, in defiance of hospital-issue, wrinkle-free polyester.

"Ha-ha," Mandi turned her head one way, then the other. Steroids had shrunk the mass that grew from her nose but not the one in her throat. Her voice sounded nasal and muffled, as if she held a hot potato in her mouth.

"Really," I said. "You look awesome, now that that thing isn't hanging out of your nose."

"I'm seeing double," Mandi said. She turned to me.

Something was wrong with her eye. Between 8 a.m. and now, at 6:30 p.m., her left eye had shifted. It veered off to the side, independently seeking the far wall.

"I see two of you," Mandi said. "And it's not funny."

Two hours later, Mandi lay in the CT scanner. A new cauliflower was sprouting from her left eye socket. It pushed her eyeball forward. The old tumor that grew down her throat now rested against her larynx; her airway was in danger of obstruction. It was highly unusual that a definitive diagnosis could not be made, but it was clear, for Mandi's sake, the oncologists could wait no longer. They made their best guess and concocted an ad lib chemotherapy regimen. After one more biopsy, they began dripping poison into her veins.

The next afternoon, my pager erupted. The message flashed STAT. I found Mandi in her room, vomiting blood on the floor. Her mother stood in the corner. Rigid. Horrified. I grabbed a trash can. I held it beneath Mandi's chin. I wrapped one arm around her shoulders and drew her against me. We sat side by side on her bed; her heaving, me holding. Mandi hemorrhaged from her new biopsy site and lost more than half her blood volume that day. I held her.

Mandi required surgery to stop her bleeding. She emerged from the OR with an endotracheal tube in place to secure her airway. She was admitted to the ICU, an action that removed me from her care team. But by that point, the artificial constraints of hospital services meant nothing to me. I cared about Mandi in a way that was different from the distant, objective way I had been taught to care about patients. I cared about Mandi as a girl, as her parents' daughter. I cared about her as a friend. Nothing could change that.

I showed up in Mandi's room every morning. And when I could finagle a lunch break, and in the middle of the night when I was on call. Mandi couldn't speak because the breathing tube parted her vocal cords, but she could write. Her brother had brought her a slate, and a carton of chalk, and neither left Mandi's lap. She wrote things like, *What is happening? When can I go home? Am I going to die?* I had no answers, nor did anyone else.

Despite chemotherapy, the tumor in Mandi's left eye socket grew. Fast. Within days her eyeball was in danger of being completely ejected. Mandi was transported by ambulance once a day to undergo emergency radiation therapy at the University of Washington. Just as that tumor began to shrink, another one began pushing her right eye out of its socket.

Two weeks after her ICU admission and nearly five weeks after she came to the hospital, Mandi wrote on her slate: *I need a shower.*

"You have a tube in your lungs," I said. "You can't take a shower."

The statement sat there between us.

"Your nurse can clean you up," I said. "Or your mom."

Mandi wrote: *I NEED A SHOWER, NOW!!!* And then she flung the slate like a Frisbee against the wall.

Mandi was driven, and she possessed a determination, even as her body was being hijacked by disease, that could not be ignored. I received permission from her nurse and then she and I got to work.

There was one bathroom in the ICU, intended for patient families. I helped Mandi out of bed. Both of her eyes bulged now and she was bald from the chemotherapy no one believed was working against the cancer no one could diagnose. She was so weak she couldn't walk without holding on to my arm. By the time we made it to the bathroom, she was panting. The tube hung from her mouth and she drooled around it. She clutched the bathroom doorknob in one hand, my shoulder with the other. It was the first time I'd seen Mandi cry.

I held Mandi from behind as she adjusted the taps. Then— determined, beyond any reasonable expectation, to do it herself—she shooed me into the hall. I leaned against the wall. I watched nurses pushing gurneys and wheelchairs, wiping down mattresses, rolling racks of sterile instruments, emesis basins, and bedpans. I never felt more unlike a doctor than during those fifteen minutes I spent stationed outside the ICU bathroom.

Medicine had failed Mandi; it could not cure her, it could not even slow the progression of her disease. If I had done anything to help Mandi, it was not because I held medical degrees, it was only because I had strayed from the confines of a physician. That day I felt like the last warm creature on a cold planet. I felt like a human. I felt like a friend.

Six days after her shower, Mandi stopped breathing. The unnamed cancer had invaded her liver and lungs, her intestines and stomach. It seemed the more chemo she received, the faster the tumors grew. Mandi's neck bulged, her tongue bulged, her belly bulged. Mandi went blind. She scrawled on her slate, *I don't want people to see me.* She wrote, *Don't let them come.* She wrote, *Thank you.*

Mandi had been in the hospital six weeks. It was early April. I was sitting on the edge of her bed when she died.

I remember a late night trip to a grocery store, in Houston, Texas. A woman in line recognized me; she was an ophthalmologist. I was a fourth-year medical student, approaching graduation. The woman said, "What are you going into?"

"Pediatrics," I said. "I'm moving to Seattle."

She shook her head, gave a little dismissive snort through her nose. "Boring," she said. "And besides, you're too smart for that. You should go into surgery."

I walked out of the market, into Houston's oppressive humidity. The dank odor of refining petroleum hung in the air. I didn't want to be a mechanic, a technician focused on splicing a body back together again. I wanted to take care of *people*. I wanted to be a physician in the ancient tradition, a physician who touched others—physically and emotionally. A physician who sought to heal, not merely to treat. I made a promise, right then, to leave medicine if ever I lost the joy of caring.

I knew nothing, at that early stage, about what that promise might demand. About the cost of fulfilling it.

I never found Pediatrics boring. I never found anything about medicine boring. On the contrary. I found people endlessly engaging. I found addressing their needs and concerns frustrating at times, but always fulfilling.

But, in the end, I couldn't sustain the effort. I found that practicing medicine, the way I felt I should practice it, was an emotional burden I couldn't carry.

I wonder, sometimes, if I would have been better off— professionally—with a little more callousness and indifference. I wonder if I might still be practicing medicine had I heeded the warnings of my teachers, had I never sat on Mandi's bed.

But for all those years afterwards—all those days I spent examining patients in the windowless rooms of a clinic, all those early mornings rounding on newborns and on kids with asthma and infections and dehydration—I never forgot her. Mandi met me around every corner, held me accountable to question my biases. She taught me to talk. She taught me I could never again hold myself distant and call myself a doctor.

The last time I saw Karen she was so thin her jeans puckered beneath her belt. Her left side was paralyzed and her speech slurred; a little spittle escaped her mouth when she spoke. She required a wheelchair to attend church and her daughters' soccer games. When I arrived, Karen wanted to take a drive in the desert. Her husband, bless him, understood our desire to be alone. He helped her into the car, I fastened her seatbelt. Karen asked me to tip her to the right so she could lean against the passenger door, and I did.

We drove for miles through winter-starved mesquite, bare thorny branches like black claws against the pale sky. We drove into the hills, cluttered with shattered rock and clusters of prickly pear. It was my seventh visit over the course of Karen's illness and I knew it would be my last. She knew it, too.

That day we shared silence and landscape—we always had. But we also talked, and touched. Karen's fatal illness left her no room for emotional guardedness; my life experience—forever altered by Mandi— had brought me to the same place.

We talked that day of big things. Of our unbounded love for our kids, of our deep and complicated love for our husbands, of our convoluted love for our parents; we talked of the love we felt for so many good friends and of the love we felt for one another. We talked of the dream of mountains that brought us together and of the most beautiful places in the world we had seen. We talked about our spiritual beliefs and agonized over why, it seemed, God chose to heal some people and not others. We talked about how fighting death appeared futile, yet giving up was not an option. We talked about kicking a soccer ball and how it was impossible now but what about in heaven, and was heaven real and if it wasn't how in the world could Karen die without knowing?

And then we decided there is no knowing. There is only faith. Faith that children will remember, that children will grow, that husbands will mourn and love again. Faith that whatever the unknown turns out to be, it will be known, and that those two words, *will be*, constitute all the hope in the world.

On the way home, Karen needed to pee. I pulled into a gas station.

"I can't do this alone," she said.

"I'll help you in."

"No, I mean, I really can't do it," Karen pressed her forehead against her window. "I can't get up off the toilet. I can't deal with my jeans."

We held on to each other and headed to the restroom. The door swung shut behind us and I unfastened her belt. I pulled down her jeans, then her underpants. I lowered her onto the toilet. Then I stepped outside and leaned against the cinder-block wall. It was late February in West Texas and the wind felt like an icy blowtorch. Tumbleweeds massed against a barbed wire fence. Dust tornadoed into the cactus. A white plastic grocery bag, caught in the mesquite, whipped like a torn sail. Karen kicked the door to let me know she was finished.

I lifted and braced her against the wall until she was balanced on her right foot, then I pulled up her pants. "Jesus," I said, "if anyone ever told me at Baylor I would be doing this, I would have said they were out of their mind."

"It's insane," Karen said. "But I'm glad it's you."

And then she caught the toe of her shoe on the bathroom threshold. She lurched forward. I lunged and grabbed at her waist. She had lost so much weight she wasn't heavy, but the momentum of her half-paralyzed body in free fall was immense. In that split second of time I knew I couldn't hold her, I knew I had done all I could do.

But, somehow, Karen didn't fall. We stood there a minute, I with both arms clutching her waist, she with her left foot stuck in the door. We shimmied backwards and sideways and stood a minute more. The plastic bag tore itself loose and skidded over the pavement in our direction.

"Thank you," Karen said.

I pulled her bald head into the crook of my neck. Her skin smelled faintly musty, like damp dirt after a desert rainstorm, like the wind when all the leaves have fallen from the trees.

Call it disillusionment. Call it cynicism. Call it burnout. Call it anything you like, but in the end, call it human. Mandi tied my professional life and my personal life in an inextricable knot. Ten years after Karen's death, twenty years after Mandi's, I left medicine for something new.

The burden of leaving has been nearly as great as the burden of staying. I miss the drama, I miss the mundane. I miss the challenge, the camaraderie, and the privilege of connection.

It is a shame I could not find a way to reconcile the personal and the professional. Part of me wants to believe it could have been different. But I'm not sure that is true. My husband, a teacher of medical school graduates, tells me he receives young doctors every year who are still taught the same things. Taught to believe it is unacceptable to sit on a patient's bed. That comforting touch is to be avoided. That compassion for patients cannot include affection. As a physician, it is difficult to turn one's back on that which is taught with such authority. Yet, for me, it was as difficult—in the end, impossible—to ignore my own heart.

All this being said, to leave the profession to which I dedicated twenty-five years of my life was a sacrifice. But what I have gained far outweighs anything I have lost. Mandi taught me to talk. Karen taught me to touch. In medicine, everything in between felt like a fire, deliberately set.

THIRTY MINUTES CLOSER

Leah E. Mintz

It was four o'clock in the morning. I was lying under a white sheet in the cardiothoracic intensive care unit with tears rolling down my cheeks, the cadence of the monitors drifting in from the dim hallway. Some of the least stable patients in the hospital were splayed out on beds in the rooms around me—where the rhythmic din was the only evidence they were still alive—but I thought I was worse off than any of them, the only one in there without a monitor or machine to keep me going, to save my life.

How did this happen? How did I end up in an ICU bed, on call for the first time, surrounded by bodies, people hovering at the edge of a crevasse, attached to tubes and wires in an effort to keep them from falling to their deaths? Some of these patients had open chest incisions so the heart could be massaged if it decided to give up the fight. The wounds were covered with translucent, mustard-colored dressings to keep them sterile. The struggling heart was visible through the sticky wrap, laboriously pushing blood to the pale, starved, motionless body lying there. The bodies were always swollen, their faces unrecognizable even to those who loved them. To me, they were unrecognizable even as people. They were the embodiment of a dream I'd had many times. A car crash in the middle of the night. Crushed and bloodied bodies strewn across the road. And me—faced with the expectation that I will know what to do. I am instead horrified by the gore, immobilized by fear.

I lifted my brand-new pager from the bedside table to check the time: 0411. The alarm on the pager was set for 4:30. Morning rounds would begin at 6 a.m. The chief resident would escort the attending around the unit to each bedside, residents and medical students scurrying along behind like ducklings, so that I, their dutiful intern, could tell them everything they wanted to know about all these patients. I wondered if four-thirty was early enough. Gently, I placed the beeper back down, afraid to jostle it into paging me. Earlier in the day, I had tried to sneak away to a phone so I could hear a comforting voice from my former life and got six pages within about sixty seconds—one from a nurse asking what to do about a patient's low potassium level. I said maybe we should give him some potassium, unless she knew of any reason we shouldn't. She didn't, she said. How much did I want to give? "How much do you usually give," I asked her idiotically.

I wiped my wet cheek, trying not to move the noisy plastic liner on the mattress beneath me. The person sleeping in the next bed was the only person in the world who could possibly save me, and I couldn't let him see my despair. He was the cardiothoracic fellow, training to be a cardiothoracic surgeon, his general surgery residency behind him. To me, he was like a TV character, sitting casually on the counter at the nurses' station, laughing with the other fellows, looking good in his scrubs. I hated him for that, but mostly I hated him for not understanding, for being so far removed from being an intern that he no longer remembered what it was like to be scared and alone. I hated him, and I wanted to crawl under the covers with him and put his arms around me. I wanted him to carry me away from the wreckage. I could get up right now, leave my ID badge and white coat by the bed, walk past the nurses' station and down the stairs to the main level, push open the hospital doors, and step out into the balmy night air, into a world where I used to live.

But I couldn't walk out. I couldn't do that any more than I could go unplug the ventilator breathing for the patient in the next room.

On the first day of medical school, one of the professors, formal and self-satisfied, stood behind a clunky wood podium and told an auditorium full of scared men and women that we wouldn't all make it through to the end; it would be too hard for some of us. But I did make it. In first-year anatomy class, I met my cadaver, named her, and dissected her. I never told anyone I was thinking about death or about the guilt I felt for cutting off her body parts so I could learn about the brachial plexus or the pancreatic duct. Looking down at her rubbery face, breathing in the foul-smelling preservative, I thought I must have come here to face my worst fears. Death. Failure. Humiliation. And maybe the worst of it: the loss of control, always waiting to be called to someone else's disaster, waiting to be seen for what you fear you are— an imposter, a fraud. This was my nightmare come to life, bodies all around, expectation staring me down.

I made it through the first live patients too, the ones who know your interviewing and prodding are superfluous and inconsequential, and worse, the ones who think you know something that could actually help them—their questions and hopeful glances tying your guts in a knot. I survived all the tests, the endless memorization, the crushing pressure. I got As in all my classes but one, and matched into a competitive surgical residency. Our attending liked to tell us we were the cream of the crop, although he usually asked us why, then, we were doing such a supremely pitiful job. I thought I'd done everything you were supposed to do to be ready for what would come next.

In medical school, you can make a bunch of mistakes without causing much trouble for anyone other than yourself. But residency was different. A month or so after my cardiothoracic ICU rotation, I was robotically completing the tasks on my cluttered scut list for the urology service when I realized I had confused two of the patients, thereby removing someone's surgical staples too soon. No real harm done—that was clear to me later—but I was mortified and called the attending surgeon to confess my sin. "I've committed an egregious error," I said melodramatically, and for the remainder of my residency he never made eye contact with me again. To him—even five years later, when I was chief resident for Head and Neck Surgery—I would always be the intern who screwed up. And who can blame him? Real people could get hurt and doctors' reputations were on the line.

When I was in my fifth year of residency, taking one of the junior residents through a tracheostomy on a cancer patient, one of us—I can't remember who—performed a routine maneuver using a hemostat to spread the tissue next to the trachea. The sudden, massive hemorrhage was like someone had turned on a faucet full force somewhere deep in the wound. I knew full well that it would take only a minute or two for the patient to bleed out and die right in front of us, the other resident and I standing there frozen, staring down at the bloody mess. I heard myself yelling for lap pads and heavy clamps and saw my gloved hands frantically pressing gauze into the wound, trying to tamponade the injured vessel. I watched with mounting horror as the bleeding overwhelmed even two large suctions and multiple hands applying all the pressure we could manage. In the end, one blindly placed clamp stopped the exsanguination and the patient survived, but not without the vascular surgeons being called in, an intraoperative angiogram revealing the patient's abnormal vascular anatomy—her subclavian artery tethered up into her neck next to the trachea—and the vascular surgeons performing an ilio-axillary bypass in order to restore blood flow to her arm.

Had I made a mistake? I don't know. I was never blamed for causing this crazy, almost incomprehensible sequence of events. In fact, for the remainder of my training I was affectionately teased for being the only resident ever to do a tracheostomy that required rerouting the arterial blood supply from the groin to prevent the arm from dying. Nonetheless, whether I erred or not, I was graphically, publicly reminded that one wrong turn and death, humiliation, failure—all that I'd come here to face—could broadside you without warning and do you in.

Throughout my residency I was told, "If you don't have complications, you're not operating enough." I don't think anyone really believes this; no one wants complications to happen on their watch. Of course, no one wants bad things to happen to patients, but in the hierarchy of medical training, what you really don't want is to be blamed for any bad things done by someone else. So, if all goes well, the interns will make it through the year with their marionette strings untangled and the people around them—patients and co-residents alike—unscathed. At least that's what it looks like from above: the perfect intern, goofy smile painted on her emotionless face, arms and legs being guided through the motions somewhat awkwardly, never complaining about the strings. But from eyes peering out from beneath a hospital sheet in the half-dark night, the view is obscured by emotion, blurred by tears.

"This is a lonely place," I thought, my eyelids drifting closed. I could see myself, earlier in the day, running through the doors into the unit, eyes wide and scanning, trying to figure out why the nurse on the phone had told me with irritation, or maybe anxiety, to come right away. The noise in the unit was more urgent than usual and people were everywhere. Someone was crashing, that much was obvious from the cloud of hornets circling one of the beds. I just wasn't sure what they wanted me to do about it. Then I saw one of the ICU nurses facing out from the crowd, beckoning me toward her, holding open a sterile gown for me to walk into. The dread started to move through me, like time-lapsed images of fungus spreading over a dead leaf. My arms rose out in front of me, suspended from above by their strings, waiting for the gown to be positioned. Someone put a cap over my hair and wrapped a mask around my face. They ushered me into the room to the bedside, next to the body, the patient, the person who was dying. "This is ridiculous," I thought. "I'm totally out of my league and everyone in here knows it. Only they're not doctors, and since I was the first one to show up, I have to do this."

Peel off the dressing, the nurse urged. *Cup your hands around the heart. Squeeze. Try to get the pressure up. Not so fast, just steady.* Everyone stared up at the monitor as if the patient were up there, hanging from the ceiling. *Not getting better. Charging,* she yelled, and crammed the paddles into my hands. *Clear!* The body lurched off the bed and back down with a thud. The flailing heart was in my hands again, rocking sluggishly back and forth. Everything I'd ever learned became irrelevant. This oddly shaped muscle seemed to have a mind of its own; it contracted to its own rhythm and I had no idea how it did that. I did my best to help it along, reaching intrusively into the chest, imposing the will of the bedside throng. We were shoulder to shoulder, layered two or three deep, undulating around the body like waves lapping at the hull of a marooned boat. And with each breath from the ventilator, the patient's lungs inflated, enveloping my hands in bags of tiny, pink pockets of air. It was a dance, a rhythmic chant to the gods. And so it went. Me in a haze, watching from somewhere outside myself as medications were injected, nurses yelled and scribbled notes, my hands applied the paddles and massaged the heart, until gradually the pitch of the oxygen saturation monitor started to rise. The patient's swollen face lost its blue hue and went back to off-white, adorned with tiny drops of sweat. He had been resuscitated, brought back from the mouth of the crevasse by the cardiothoracic ICU team and their puppet.

If I were a TV character playing opposite my handsome CT fellow, I would have pulled off my mask and cap, let my shiny hair fall gracefully around my perfect face, and basked in the self-satisfaction of it all. A life had been saved, and everyone out there in TV-Land would be happy to give me the credit for it. But I knew I was merely playing a part, a body filling a spot, holding someone's heart, someone's life, in my hands. Somewhere inside, my own heart wobbled. My own life, the one I had before this, had slipped away, and I seemed to have lost myself somehow, too. This is how it works, we were told: you sacrifice yourself for a few grueling years in exchange for being spit out at the other end, re-sculpted into a surgeon. You give up your autonomy and agree to get carried along like this, until slowly, bit by bit, you start to know stuff other people need. I should have been happily answering pages, skipping down the hallway to offer my cheerful assistance. That's what my TV character would have done, after all. But when it comes right down to it, when someone else decides when you eat and sleep, being needed isn't fun.

There are catch phrases in medicine, perfected by the people who call you from the emergency room to lure you out from under the blanket on the call-room bed. "Posterior epistaxis." That's one of their favorites. Call the Head and Neck resident for a nosebleed in the ER and say it's a posterior bleed. It almost never is. A true posterior nosebleed from one of the large vessels in the back of the nose requires a special kind of pack, so the Head and Neck resident has to go check it out. But they're rare. Most nosebleeds, even severe ones, come from the smaller vessels toward the front of the nose and should be within the purview of the competent emergency room physician. So when the ER resident tells you there's a patient with a posterior bleed, it generally means, "I don't want to deal with this anymore and I don't want you to finagle your way out of taking care of it for me."

"Mobile midface" is another one. Not as devious and comes up less frequently, but those two words let you know you'll be getting out of bed to see a trauma patient with facial fractures. One night late in my residency, the chief resident for General Surgery called me from the emergency room and said, "The midface is mobile," eliciting the all-too-familiar flip of anxiety and resentment in my stomach. This most likely meant I'd be up the rest of the night, examining the patient, writing my consult report, waiting for the results of the CT scan. I stayed under the covers until I admitted to myself that the turmoil in my head wasn't relaxing anyway, and then wrenched my body from the bed.

Busy emergency rooms that see lots of trauma are noisy places, full of drama and, if you're in the mood for it, excitement. I wasn't in the mood. I traipsed over to the patient lying on the gurney in Trauma 1 and looked down at his face. "What have you done to yourself?" I asked him. He didn't answer. He was intubated, sedated. This probably meant he had other serious injuries elsewhere in the body, unless they thought he needed airway protection because of his facial fractures. But that didn't make sense because his face didn't look so bad. He had some abrasions, some small lacerations, but there wasn't a lot of swelling and the contours of his face looked fine. For the midface to be mobile, the fractures have to be severe enough that the upper jaw is separated from the rest of the skull. You test for this by holding the head still with one hand, grasping the upper teeth with the other, and then seeing if you can move the upper jaw around. I tried this and the teeth did move. But there was no blood and too little resistance. I took a closer look and then removed the full upper denture from the patient's mouth. There were no fractures. The midface was mobile because the patient hadn't glued in his denture that morning.

I looked across the room at the General Surgery chief resident. He was a jovial guy and I liked him. He looked back at me holding the denture up in the air and a wide grin slowly spread across his face. And then he started laughing. His high-pitched, infectious laugh grew louder and more unruly, until the sound of it drowned out the other noise and it was all I could hear. I started laughing too, reluctantly at first, but then gratefully, recklessly, until our laughter was a cacophonous duet, irreverent and out of place.

Maybe being needed could be fun, but that first night in the cardiothoracic unit, it wasn't another doctor who needed me. I needed me—to see the humor, to see my own value, to be open to camaraderie, to remember why this work was important. But mostly, to feel happy. Lying there, staring at the ICU ceiling with countless nights in the hospital ahead of me, the laughter was too far away to hear over the sound of the monitors, and the happiness ahead too dim for me to see. I reached for the pager and looked at the time: 0429. I closed my eyes, took a deep, slow breath, and heard the alarm sound.

THE CLEVEREST DOCTOR

Clint Morehead

> Doctors would prove cleverest if, beginning in childhood,
> in addition to learning the art, they should be familiar
> with very many and very bad bodies and should themselves
> suffer all diseases and not be quite healthy by nature.
> —Plato, *The Republic*

I.

I don't know what it is to be sick. I have caught a cold, as everyone has, endured a stomachache, contracted chickenpox from a kindergarten classmate and boast a scar to prove it. I have had strep throat once and been given a shot to make it go away. And I have had pneumonia, my mom tells me, followed by a stint of asthma that lasted a couple years.

Neither of these two afflictions can I remember. I can't say I've seen much more than that.

I was not a floppy baby, nor was my heart the shape of a boot. My feet never resembled clubs, my spine was never bamboo-shaped on an X-ray, my legs never bowed. I'm sure my parents were delighted, twenty-six years ago, to find me, having just been toweled dry for the first time, my Apgars counted and recorded, to be endowed with ten fingers and ten toes, a face of normal proportion, and a strong cry. Though they couldn't see them, each of my cells bore the correct number of chromosomes, no errant bands, no fragile Xs. My pediatrician with his baby stethoscope, at some point, found my heart standing by in its usual location, thumping smoothly and evenly like a bird's, without murmur, without rub. And through stories, I know that he eventually took a look at me, then at my parents, sized us up, and announced, "He's gonna be tall. Six foot two, at least." And I remember my dismay, sixteen years later, when I realized that, most likely, I had peaked. I had reached five foot ten two years earlier, and that was it; I've been there ever since.

Otherwise, nature has been good to me. I never found myself burdened with a congenital megacolon, and to my knowledge, the tiny foot processes of my glomeruli have never been effaced. I've searched my fingertips for the illusive lesions of Janeway, spots of Roth, and nodes of Osler, but have come up empty. My fingers themselves have not assumed the shape of a swan's neck, and I would be astonished to see that my lower esophagus is tight and narrow, the rest ballooned, resembling a bird's beak. The fluid surging through my vessels, as far as I know, has always been free of schistocytes, spherocytes, target cells, sickle cells, Reed-Sternberg cells, even Gaucher's cells. The last time I checked my skin, for the life of me, I could not find a single café au lait spot. I don't have a port wine stain either, though I had a friend in college who was born with one. It covered half of his face, and for the longest time, that salient bright red splotch was the only way I could distinguish him from his twin brother.

My ophthalmologist has never let on that she's found a cherry red spot on my macula, so I have no reason to believe I have one. I have never produced impressive sputum into a Kleenex, nothing that meets the criteria for "currant jelly." I would be astonished to learn that deep inside, I have a chocolate cyst, a honeycomb lung, or a nutmeg liver, all of which sound a bit appetizing, but in truth, I know I'm lucky not to have them. My basement membranes have always held strong. My pancreas, parathyroid, and pituitary all work the way they should. I am not a blue bloater or a pink puffer. I am not female, fat, fertile, or forty—the risk factors for gallstones. I have never felt the onset of ptosis, miosis, and anhidrosis, or the sudden loss of control of one side of my face, one side of my mouth, a hand, an arm, a leg, or any combination thereof. I do not know the frustration of searching for a single word that with all my strength I just cannot say. I do not know the agonizing electric shocks you get with trigeminal neuralgia. I have never felt Hammon's crunch. I have never lost control of my bladder after having it my whole life. I have never fought in a war and then found myself home, alone, searching for just one person who *gets* me, who's seen what I've seen, who's done what I've done. I have never had a whole life laid out before me, only to find one day that I have tiny spots in my brain that sometimes make me see flashes of light, that other times make my fingers tingle or my voice slur or my right leg go limp for an hour. I have never had epilepsy. I have never had cancer. I have never watched someone I love die.

II.

This week, one of my patients is a doctor. I have been assigned to follow him and to learn something from him, as is the routine of a medical student. I am a fourth-year now, rotating a second time through the cancer ward at University Hospital. He has malignant melanoma, stage IV, meaning that it has spread to remote parts of his body—the brain and pelvis to be exact. He is here for chemo.

I enter his room early each morning, check that his vital signs and labs haven't wandered above or below the normal range, make sure that he's getting all his medications, that he isn't in pain, that he can still drink water without getting nauseated, that his bowel movements are regular. Then I listen to his heart, lungs, and abdomen. I feel for pulses in his feet, squeeze his ankles to see if there is any swelling. I offer anything else he needs before I leave.

I first met him on a Monday morning. The resident on the oncology service suggested that I follow him, not necessarily so that I could see firsthand the havoc that this particularly toxic chemotherapy regimen bestows, but because the resident learned from the patient's wife that a third-year medical student, on his family medicine rotation in rural Kentucky, had been assigned to stay with this doctor, in his house with his family, and to shadow him for four weeks. The doctor had been looking forward to accommodating this student for months. In rural Kentucky, students are hard to come by, but doctors, the best kind, no matter where they are, are inherently teachers, and this doctor wanted to teach more than anything. Upon being diagnosed with melanoma, my patient was immediately scheduled for brain surgery and chemotherapy, an extremely harsh treatment plan that would require time, lots of it. He knew he needed to take an extended leave of absence, and, dismayed, he knew that this would conflict with his student's rotation. In light of learning this, the resident, hoping that in some way I could assume the role of that student, asked me if I would visit him in the mornings.

It is heartbreaking to watch someone go through chemotherapy, especially the kind they give melanoma patients. I had, in fact, followed many patients with metastatic melanoma by this time, and the doctor fell victim to its toxic side effects just as everyone else had. After one day, his skin flushed bright red, his heart began to race, accompanied by uncontrollable sweating and diarrhea, which would not abate until the course of treatment was over. The levels of several essential components of his blood began to fluctuate. The white blood cells shot up to alarming levels that would make it appear as though he had leukemia, but in reality this was the response expected for this type of chemotherapy, which stimulates the immune system. We kept a close watch on his temperature. Soon the platelets, heralds of blood clots, would drop, and he ran the risk of sudden bleeding. Once they dropped dangerously low, and we had to hold one of the components of the chemo, the cisplatin. The potassium and magnesium would inevitably decrease as well, due to the chemo's effects on the kidneys, so we replaced them accordingly lest a deadly heart arrhythmia take our doctor away.

I learned that he was a family practice physician whose wife had driven him all the way to Louisville from London, Kentucky, about two and a half hours away, and five days later, would drive him back home. She stationed herself in a recliner that doubled as a bed for family members who wanted to stay overnight. Over the course of the week, she would leave the room only once or twice a day to buy herself a meal in the basement cafeteria, then return promptly to eat beside her husband. The attached restroom allowed her to stay near, even for those brief intermissions. Family pictures, I noticed, were arranged upon the sill of the picture window spanning the entire far side of the room, the blinds drawn shut for the duration of their stay. The photos showed kids smiling with their healthy grandfather. There was also an 8 x 10-inch photograph of a house, ranch-style, situated on what looked to be a few acres of land. I could only imagine that it was theirs, and that seeing it brought them comfort.

When I enter, the room is dark, lit only by the lighting from the hall. I don't bother to turn on the lights. The doctor has dark gray hair, disheveled and flattened against the pillow. Covering his face are fine whiskers, gray also; he appears not to have shaven for a few days. He is wearing a hospital gown that is falling off his right shoulder. He is curled, in his bed, to one side with one leg tucked underneath a quilt they brought from home, the other leg out. He has contorted himself into a modified fetal position, chin tucked down, knees and hips flexed inward. He and his wife are both sleeping. With hesitation I wake them; they are happy to see me.

As I do the necessary exam and ask the necessary questions, he and his wife ask me about myself. They want to know where I'm planning on doing my residency. I tell them that I'm thinking about staying here because I like taking care of patients who come from where I grew up, but I say that I'm still looking around and have interviews scheduled all over the country, as most medical students do during the fall and winter of their fourth year. I'm not sure whether they just assumed or whether the resident said something, but the doctor and his wife are under the impression that I am going to become a family medicine doctor, even though in reality, I am applying for programs in internal medicine, which is different. I don't correct them. The doctor names several family medicine doctors whom he thinks I may have worked with, but none of them are familiar to me. "It may help you if you meet some of them," he says. "You might have a better chance of getting hired if you have some people on the inside who know you." I nod in acquiescence.

His skin feels as if he's been baking in an oven. I nervously press my stethoscope against his chest, knowing well that he knows more than I do about listening to someone's heart. I make sure I listen in all four locations to hear all four valves: aortic, pulmonary, tricuspid, mitral. On the last one, he moves my stethoscope slightly to the left, wanting to know if I can hear it better there. I can. Next, I listen to his lungs. When I finish the front of his body, he automatically lifts himself up from his bed without my asking so I can hear the lower lobes of his lungs through his back. I extend my arm for him to use to pull himself up. The sheets underneath are soaking wet. He lies back down, and I palpate his abdomen and watch his face for a grimace, indicating pain. He has none.

"Aren't you going to ask my history?" he says. I haven't taken a full history this morning because the resident had already completed it the day before when I was in Alabama interviewing for a residency position there. "They already did that," his wife says. "He's just checking up on you." I can tell the doctor is not completely lucid. Still, I say, "You're right, I didn't get your history." I take a seat beside his bed. "Why don't you tell me your story."

I listen to him explain all that he has been through over the past seven months. He tells me about getting diagnosed and the various specialists who evaluated him. He tells me about the surgery to remove a large portion of skin on his back that contained the cancer. He describes the way they kept him awake during his brain surgery to remove the one lesion they saw on his MRI. Then he tells me how later, from another MRI that was taken a few months after the surgery, more lesions were found, and as a result, he was scheduled for whole-brain radiation. In the meantime, every six weeks, he and his wife travel to Louisville for rounds of this chemotherapy. "It's been a tough year," is all I can say. I ask if there's anything else he needs, and I back myself into the hall and quietly shut the door.

III.

I spent a month in Paducah last summer with an oncologist who told me that ten years after he started practicing medicine he dropped the white coat, realizing that it intimidated his patients; five years after that, he stopped wearing a tie. Eight months before I shadowed him, he had fallen from a ladder while repairing his barn and had broken his back. He had just returned from six months of leave but still walked with a noticeable limp. He told me he'd try to continue working, though he anticipated the back pain would make it difficult, and he foresaw himself retiring within the year.

I remember my White Coat Ceremony, just days before I opened my first medical textbook, as if it were yesterday. It's been nearly four years now. I remember seeing my classmates for the first time, not knowing their names or anything about them. I remember standing on a stage, a doctor I'd never met before ungracefully twisting me into the white coat as an auditorium of faces watched. I remember thinking, "This is it. I'm here. I've finally made it." Then, two years later, on the eve of my first clinical rotation, the day that every first- and second-year medical student can't wait to see, that same white coat ended up in my parents' washer with a multicolored retractable pen in its pocket. Forty-five minutes later it emerged a tie-dyed mess. I ordered a new one immediately.

Two years after that, just weeks from graduation, and my second white coat is far from white. It is now dirty and soiled and worn; threads appear daily from the edges of its collar, the seams around its pockets, the folds at its wrists. I have trained myself to watch for them, and when I find them, I trim my white coat like an old dog. A mysterious stain around the collar refuses to disappear, as do others. A faint brown smudge upon the left shoulder is what remains of a peanut butter and jelly sandwich I ate one night on call. An interrupted black stripe across the back came from my bike's chain brushing against its folds, my white coat wadded up into a pile of fabric on the floor of my car's trunk. This is where it spends most of its nights, for the prospect of wandering the halls in a coatless state of dishabille, disrobed as in a nightmare, I don't want to imagine. So for safety I leave it in the car, outside and alone. The coat knows the night better than I: the winter's cold, the summer's heat, the sounds, the darkness. One night someone broke into my car, ripped the stereo out of the dash, stole several CDs, but left the white coat. The following morning, like every other morning, I retrieved it from the trunk, shook out its wrinkles, brushed off the fragments of dried leaves, and went about my business.

On its right cuff, a spattering of rusty spots is all that remains of a splay of venous blood flicked from a catheter during a botched attempt to place a central line. A yellowish mark underneath the third button is ascetic fluid from a tap done in the ER at four o'clock one morning. My resident, I remember, warned that the patient was a screamer, and like clockwork, she let out a blood-curdling shriek that echoed through the ER before the needle had even touched her skin. Eventually, I learned that the tap had shown a severe infection, and over the course of the following week the patient was transferred to the ICU and slowly drifted away, yet another victim of drugs and alcohol. The second button from the top is missing. A year ago, my team and I were rounding in a patient's room, the attending and the patient discussing something serious, when out of the blue the button took a dive, as if to say, "That's it. I've had enough!" and leapt to its symbolic death, tinging against the floor before coming to rest under the hospital bed, raising the room's sobriety to levity, my face red with chagrin.

My white coat carries an arsenal of equipment that weighs it down. The right outer pocket holds a mini-clipboard. Clipped in are notecards containing jotted-down patients' lab values, vital signs, physical exams, and scribbled notes of article titles that my attending and residents want me to read. My black pager, dormant now, and a pinlight are clipped to the inside of this pocket. A reflex hammer has fallen deep, as well as some pens and a bottle of hand sanitizer. Inside the left outer pocket are reference materials: *The Massachusetts Gen-*

eral Hospital Handbook of Internal Medicine, which I didn't purchase until just this year because of its high price, and the *Sanford Guide to Antimicrobial Therapy*, just as useful, given to me for free. Wrapped together with a rubber band are two items that my surgery attending, Dr. Pierce, scolded me one day for not having with me: "A pocket pharmacopeia and a pen," she said from behind her surgical mask. "Every student who ever scrubs with me must have these items, or I'll kick them out," she said in a Viola Swamp–esque tone. She required us to write the post-op notes so I carried the *Maxwell Quick Medical Reference Guide* as well, which explains how to do this. I remember my classmate Jordan, who couldn't stand Dr. Pierce, showing up to the OR one day with the full-sized version of the pharmacopeia, neon orange and covered in plastic. "That's never going to fit in your scrubs' pocket, you know," Dr. Pierce informed her. Then Jordan, looking her straight in the eye, the rest of their faces covered completely by masks (there was no hiding), spitefully stuffed it in with all her effort—stitches exploding from the seams, the unmistakable sound of ripping fabric tearing through the air of the OR, louder than the buzz of electrocautery and the constant beeping of the ventilator, she made it fit. These two small references, the pharmacopeia and the *Maxwell*, and a pen, remain bound together, not because I use them in tandem, but as a relic, a reminder of Dr. Pierce and how I not only passed but survived, as did Jordan.

On the inside is another pocket, and there I keep my stethoscope. I was told once by an eighty-six-year-old internist that a stethoscope should never be worn around the neck because, he said, "it's pretentious and looks stupid." His comment reminded me of a friend who grew up in my neighborhood whose mother, a nurse, would wear her stethoscope to her son's swim meets, and at least once that I knew of, to the grocery store.

Occasionally I see people wearing their white coats in public for no particular reason except, presumably, to show them off. My friends and I roll our eyes at them, knowing what fools they must be to wear what we know is the most incommodious garment in our wardrobe, only to turn heads. "I wish they'd just give us tool belts," said Megan. "I'd keep my pharmacopeia in a holster."

I can't stand wearing my white coat within the hospital, let alone outside it. All of the books and notes weigh it down, causing it to flip and flop uncontrollably as I walk down the halls, giving me the appearance of a rodeo clown, drawing more attention than I could ever need or want. The pockets inevitably get caught—in drawers or binders, on ventilator knobs—either jerking me backward or knocking something over, such as a patient's chart, spraying its pages and dividers all over the floor on impact. Even the stethoscope has its ingenious ways of harassing me, as it did last week on a packed elevator when it attached itself to the curly white hair of an elderly woman in a wheelchair.

I have in my mind this theoretical model of what the *cleverest* doctor should look like—a collage of clippings, taped and rubber-cemented together from parts of everyone I've met over the past four years, a Frankenstein creature of sorts—and he doesn't wear a white coat. He is not your stereotypical doctor. He owns a stethoscope, carried somewhere out of sight, retrieved only when needed. When his eyes come in contact with yours, you know at once that you are the only person in his world and that looking into his gaze alone could make you well. But if you spent some time with him, an hour or so, you'd realize that he addresses everyone by name and that when faced with people he doesn't know, he still makes eye contact and says "hello" or "good morning" rather than selecting his favorite crack in the sidewalk and staring at it, out of touch. He holds his stature like a Greek ideal, the essence of salubrity, but he is seated among people of every race, culture, and ethnicity, and if you were to hear them all talking, you wouldn't be able to make out who is teaching whom. All you'd know is that everyone is learning, and this is also making them well, all of them, the Frankenstein creature included.

Glued somewhere are a hammer and nails, a box of tools, a rake, and a shovel that he uses on his monthly trips to the inner city as a volunteer to help build houses. There is also a suitcase for the week he spends each summer in eastern Kentucky screening women for breast cancer and everyone for colon cancer. In one hand he holds a book or a magazine that in no way is related to the study of medicine: the *Iliad*, perhaps, *Walden*, *The New Yorker*, or *Wired*. In the other hand, of course, is *Harrison's Manual of Medicine*. Taped to his head is a cutout of a dry sponge. He wears running shoes and has a fishing pole tucked under his shoulder. He has a guitar and a piano and a Bob Dylan CD. He knows that Sir William Osler, the father of modern medicine, quoting Richard Grosseteste, agreed that "there are three things necessary for temporal salvation—food, sleep, and a cheerful disposition," and takes this to heart.

IV.

The cancer ward of University Hospital is located on the eighth floor. A few weeks after I was assigned to take care of the doctor from London, Kentucky, Mrs. Marks came to us. Her screams echoed down the halls in three of the four directions—east, west, and south—for which this hospital's inpatient areas are named. A straight shot from the elevators brings you to Eight-South, the cancer ward. As she grew nearer, Mrs. Marks's cries, like a thunderstorm, grew louder, reverberating from the walls and desks and concrete floor, invading the other patients' rooms, curling around us at work in the nurses' station. Mrs. Marks's feet were the first we saw of her, upon a gurney rounding a soft corner built into the wall to prevent collisions, followed by the rest of her diseased body. A cursory look at her chart revealed that the woman rolling horizontally past our desk had had breast cancer for years.

The other medical student and I knew that Mrs. Marks needed help, but there were no doctors around. The nurses were waiting impatiently for orders, and, from behind the counter, I wondered what I could do. I had tried paging one of the oncology fellows to tell him to come down, that orders needed to be written, but ten minutes had passed and he hadn't called back. Then, Dr. Hensley, a palliative care doctor, stepped out from one of the rooms, sized up the situation, and asked me what I was going to do. I shrugged, unsure. Mrs. Marks needed orders for pain medicine and I couldn't write them. "Why don't you go find out what she's taking at home," Dr. Hensley said. "We can use that information to calculate what to give her here."

So I walked quickly to the room where the nurses were hooking Mrs. Marks up to an IV. I saw her there, curled under a blanket, obviously suffering, and before I could introduce myself, she looked in my direction and said, "Clint, I'm really in a lot of pain. I need some help." Immediately my brain shot into motion as it tried to figure out how in the world she could have known my name. At the same time, like a jerk of the knee, without thinking, I put my hand on her shoulder. In doing so, I was nowhere I had been before.

A couple of minutes later I remembered I had seen Mrs. Marks in an outpatient clinic a few weeks earlier. She had been in for a regular checkup. We'd chatted. She'd laughed at something I'd said. That day in the hospital, I felt ashamed I hadn't jumped to my feet as quickly as I'd wanted when I saw her wheeled in. She knew who I was, yet I had forgotten her. It's funny how patients can acquaint us with ourselves, reveal certain realities we may not otherwise face. They sometimes take the darkest parts in us and bring them to the surface. When we see these parts, we may be startled, embarrassed, ashamed, but we are also changed.

Mrs. Marks, the family physician with melanoma, the oncologist from Paducah, Dr. Hensley, my classmate from high school dying of leukemia, whom I took care of last week, and others I've encountered over the past four years have taught me that while we need intellect and knowledge to effectively diagnose and treat our patients, if we're not mindful, we'll deny the instinct to react to our patients' human needs. As full as my brain is from four years of memorizing every disease imaginable, it is something else entirely, something simple, human, that told me to jump to my feet for Mrs. Marks, if only to place a hand on her shoulder and say some comforting words. I'm convinced the cleverest doctors know this.

After telling us that doctors cannot have true knowledge of a disease without having experienced it firsthand, and therefore cannot treat it, Plato qualifies: "For I don't suppose they care for a body with a body—in that case, it wouldn't be possible for the bodies themselves ever to be, or to have been, bad—but for a body with a soul; and it's not possible for a soul to have been, and to be, bad and to care for anything well." If a doctor cares for a body with his own good soul, Plato seems to be saying, what could result but goodness? At twenty-six years old, dangerously young for a doctor, just two weeks away from having that bulky MD behind my name, a new, longer white coat placed upon my shoulders, I think maybe there is hope. Maybe it is possible for us to be good doctors and to take care of our patients well, despite having never been sick a day in our lives. To compensate, I'll fill my coat pockets with the manuals, tools, and notes I'll need to make it through the days of my residency.

In time, I suspect, my white coat will grow lighter. Most doctors

I've met who have completed their formal training wear polo shirts and khakis to work, blouses and skirts, and as long as they have a place to put a stethoscope and a ballpoint pen, they may never wear a white coat at all. It's the process of molting: those things that we see are exchanged for those we don't. The only requirement is that we live, feel, know how to balance intellect and instinct, so that we can go forth, awake, doing the best we can in the time we have.

"If we are really dying," says Thoreau, "let us hear the rattle of our throats and feel cold in the extremities; if we are alive, let us go about our business."

A MANNER OF BEING

Robert Coles

This year, William Carlos Williams has, in a strange way, come alive again. The town of Rutherford, New Jersey, just celebrated his one hundred and twenty-fifth birthday—it was one hundred and twenty-five years ago that he was born, in 1883. I first learned of him in 1949. At the time, I was attending Harvard, taking a number of English literature courses from Perry Miller—who, as it turned out, quickly became the main influence in my college career. One day, Professor Miller gave me an assignment to write an essay on the work of William Carlos Williams, who, at that time, was not particularly popular in an English department devoted to T. S. Eliot and other European and Anglo-American writers. I read Williams's poetry with a great deal of interest and wrote an essay on him as a social observer—an essay that Professor Miller urged me to send to Dr. Williams. A couple of weeks later, I got back a letter on a piece of prescription paper: *William C. Williams, MD, 9 Ridge Road, Rutherford, New Jersey.* No zip code then.

> *Dear Mr. Coles,*
>   *I have received your essay on me—not bad for a Harvard student. Please drop by if you're ever in the neighborhood . . .*

Before that note's arrival, I was not inclined to give medicine a try. I was not particularly interested in, or good at, science work, such as chemistry and physics, although I managed to get by. But I took him up on his offer, taking a train from Harvard to Rutherford. The next thing I knew, I was at Columbia University's College of Physicians and Surgeons. From there, I was able to cross the Hudson River and go on house rounds with Dr. Williams, to get to know him and learn so very much from him. Williams would say to me about the patients, "What they say helps me realize what I have to say." He was emphasizing the importance of language and, most important, human connection.

I would bring books of poetry to Anatomy laboratory. Williams had the good fortune to go from high school right to medical school; he didn't have to go to college and take a lot of premed courses. I was born too late, I guess. But Williams advised me, very bluntly, to "take the damn courses and get rid of them," saying it would teach me that I could get through something. He did acknowledge that he was not sure he would be able to or want to take that approach if he were in my shoes. My mind, heart, and soul had always belonged to literature and history—and they continued to be my companions while I struggled through medical school. I'd sit there holding *Paterson* in my hand as we were doing the dissections, reading Williams's descriptions of ordinary people. One of the anatomy professors said that I ought to take that out of the lab, that it was distracting me and wasn't of any help to me and what I was doing there. But the book stayed and so did I.

Some people are drawn to medicine out of an abstract interest in science and knowledge, but the rest of us are drawn to medicine as an aspect of healing—connecting science to human ailments and suffering and vulnerability. Literature offers insight to human nature, emotional and spiritual life, and inwardness. Writers have always helped us understand about human affairs, the human mind, the human emotional life. One can learn much from reading—about ourselves, and yes, others, such as our patients. It's important to be a scientist, but it is also important to be a scientist who knows how to listen, how to think, and how to express himself or herself as clearly as possible—to get complicated ideas across to a person who has not studied medicine but who is suffering. Articulation, whether on paper or through the spoken word, is an important aspect of medical work.

For me, Williams was a heroic figure as well as a literary figure. He had, in his own way, taken on medicine by being a loner, by doing house calls—which a lot of physicians weren't doing then, at least not in the urban areas. On our first visit we went to a home in Rutherford where Dr. Williams was attending to an ailing child whose temperature was at 104 degrees. Dr. Williams shook his head in obvious concern and prescribed antibiotics, aspirin, and cold-water baths, saying, "We'll get that fever down, and the kiddo will be okay!" I remember being so impressed; he was unpretentious, informal, and yet self-assured. Here was a proudly idiosyncratic physician and healer who went out among the people and got to know them intimately in their homes, often without accepting any money from them. He'd go into the homes of working people, and he'd sit on the floor with the children and play with them, letting them hold his neurological hammer and listen to his heart through his stethoscope.

He was a hardworking physician, one who made it his business to do documentary work similar to that done by the FSA photographers during the New Deal era of the thirties—in his case, capturing the life of people with words rather than pictures, and conveying that life to others. He walked the streets of an American city; he observed; and he wrote down what he saw and heard. Williams originally wanted to be an artist; his mind was always working visually, and he had a graphic sense of the world. He used to tell me, "Keep your eyes glued." He'd say, "Look at that, look at that." He was the most visual person I've ever met—one who really looked carefully, connecting what he saw to what he was thinking as a physician.

Once, there was a young man who had serious migraine headaches, and Dr. Williams took one look at this man's forehead and afterwards said to me, "Did you see he's getting lines in his forehead, his forehead is aging because of the stress the migraine is putting on him and that stress gets expressed through a furrowed brow." He noticed that forehead; he also noticed how tightly the man tied his necktie, and he said, "Loosen it a tiny bit." He said, "It'll make you more comfortable—you can even let go of that top button on your shirt." And then Williams undid his own tie and top button, saying, "We both can relax." Our shirts unbuttoned, our ties loosened, that patient's body relaxed, and he said to Williams, "Doc, I feel better." It was a migraine—so one thing a doctor could do was prescribe aspirin. But here was a doctor going further, trying to figure out what to do, yes, but also trying to figure out what got the attacks going.

Pretty soon I was on my own, doing the kind of work Dr. Williams did: house calls, going into homes to meet children on their territory, not in a clinic or a hospital, getting to know their lives, understanding what they went through, and then writing about it. I was struggling for a certain competence, and often thought of Dr. Williams, his way of both *being* and *doing*, his "manner of being," as the existentialists would put it. At times I could hear his voice as he explained something to a particular patient, and then took action with his stethoscope or neurological hammer, or indeed, his fountain pen and prescription pad. He was a fieldworker, and he taught me to use my medical training and experience, not only as a means of both meeting people and working with them and on their behalf, but also as a means of working on my own behalf, as a would-be observer of the human condition in certain regions and areas, in homes and neighborhoods, and then conveying the heard, the observed, the learned, to others as a writer.

Like many towns and cities, Rutherford has changed. There are places now that didn't exist back when I went there. Williams's house is still there, but he is not, nor is any member of his family. The last time that I went to Rutherford, I knocked on the door to 9 Ridge Road and met a woman who lives there now—a cardiologist and a cardiac surgeon—but she didn't know that Williams had lived there. I was, at that moment, both shocked and haunted by memories of Dr. Williams. Every time I used to go to 9 Ridge Road, to that house, I'd see him and that doctor's bag of his. I remember getting in the car and going to those homes. I remember certain places—a church here, a store there— memories and reminders of change. When he was there they didn't have places named after him, but now there's a Williams Center and a Williams Plaza. I remember going there after he died and visiting his wife, Flossie. I remember the poem she gave me, one that Williams wrote for her. It begins:

> I will sing a joyous song
> > To you, my Lady!
> On a hill the wind is blowing!
> Lady, Lady, we have stood upon the hill
> > But now I'm far
> And you are far from me
> And yet the wind is all between us blowing.

In a way, Flossie was quietly telling me through the poem how a physician works: beholden to patients, but also beholden to a particular life he or she is living—we carry our affections and loyalties with us to the rooms of our patients, so that, in a sense, personal love gets soaked into the occupational caring of the physician. I remember her handing the poem to me—a wan, sad, but spirited look on her elderly face. I remember when I walked out of there tears were in my eyes. I was a doc who once got to know an American physician who happened to write—and if I hadn't met and gone on house calls with that doctor, learned from him about human nature and human suffering and human struggles, I never would have gone to medical school. The more I got to know Dr. Williams, the more I became interested in the writer as doctor and the doctor as writer—one doc handing another along a particular professional journey.

KNOCK KNOCK

Lauren Slater

M y husband likes to collect antique medical books despite the fact that he is not a doctor. A scientist who builds giant robots, my husband, although made of carbon and stardust, dwells in worlds all silicone and steel.

I wonder if my husband's penchant for crumbling medical texts found on the shelves of dusty bookstores in Maine belies the separation he must sometimes feel from his own flesh as he daily builds bodies not human. Whatever the reason, the result is that while some children grow up learning of life's darkness on the well-trod paths of fairy tales, our children have had their own unique roadways speeding them straight to the heart of hurt, sans tollbooth or exit. Despite, or because of, this, my four-year-old son and eight-year-old daughter adore their father's antediluvian collections and nightly they drag the fat books from his shelves to their beds, snuggling in for a grand lights-out story about the gangrene girl in the eighteenth century, the syphilitic man in the blacktop hat singing to God on the gaslit streets of London, or the great knight's fevered form bled by leeches, a hero felled, his armor hung on a hook, his body on a rumpled sheet, sucklers attached from scalp to sole, dark-coated doctors standing solemnly around his bed. Perhaps my favorite image of all, however, is of the electric eel-fish and the insane lady, this illustration depicting the earliest rendition of what is now a refined psychiatric treatment: electroconvulsive shock therapy (ECT), used, in our time, for the most recalcitrant cases of depression or obsessive compulsive disorder, when all medications have failed.

ECT has had a bad rap, bringing to our collective consciousness writhing women screaming as surges of current unzip their souls and psyches. In fact, ECT, despite its little understood efficacy, is a far gentler (and more effective) process in 2008 than it was in the day of Ken Kesey's *One Flew Over the Cuckoo's Nest*, an era which was itself, while not without cruelties, still a significant step up from the eighth-century scenes in my husband's tomes. Picture the picture, the illustrations all done in dark lead. There is the long-ago beach, a single wave caught in its curve, and beyond, a sunset at once magnificent and monochrome, light leaping off the page all the more mysteriously because the illustration is entirely absent of spectrum. The half disc of the setting sun is portrayed in pencil, the rays resting on the unsettled sea, the beach a would-be white except for the yellowing pall time has pressed on the paper. The beach, we are told in the italicized caption, is in Greece, a straight stretch of sand, in the center an image that pulls your vision toward its vortex: a female sprawled in a shallow tidal pool, her hair streaming away from her face like so many snakes. Kneeling by her side, in profile, is an old man whose beard belies his wisdom. Holding hefty tongs clasping electric eels, the old man applies the furious fish to the woman's scalp, which suddenly seems, in the illustration, and now in life as well, much too thin a membrane between the clumsy mortar-made world of men and the fragile ephemera of the human's hurting dream machine. The patient weeps in the water.

Medicine is an incredible field because the body it treats is an incredible organism. The human body is filled with fluids that can be either putrid or pure. When punctured, our flesh bleeds an arctic blue that, as it exits the wound, changes color in a second so swift we cannot detect the transformation. Thus we know our blood not for the teal it truly is, but for the ruby it is not.

I like to try and guess what I will die of. After all, *something* will kill me. If I am lucky I will die, as my eight-year-old daughter says with an etiquette beyond her years, "of age," but in general I'm not lucky. I've already had cancer, or something too close to it for comfort. My blood pressure is higher than it should be. Despite the fact that I eat no animal fat, plaque has clogged my plumbing in such abundance that my own internal cholesterol factory could probably fill an ongoing assembly line of tin tubs to be later labeled "shortening" (an apt designation, for what else does Crisco do but shorten one's days on earth?). Five days ago, I noticed a pain in my thigh and assumed: *strained muscle.* Four days ago, I ceased being able to walk. Getting into my nightgown, I noticed my leg was as round and red as a cartoon's swollen sausage. The skin was hot to the touch, and even the slightest press of a pinkie, or the slowest, most melodic tickle sent spritzes of burning sparks and glinting glass pain inside my infected epidermis. By morning, the redness had made its way past my knee and was clearly on the fast track to my foot. I got myself to the clinic *quickly.* Dr. Shah was young—so young! As she wrote out my antibiotic and pain med prescriptions I asked, "Are you done with medical school or are you still a resident?" I was making small talk just to distract myself from the pain. Dr. Shah looked up. "I'm done," she said. "Done done done. I'm out in the world now," she said, and then paused for a moment, pen poised in midair, as if trying to find the right word. "Practicing," Dr. Shah finally said. "I'm in the real world now. Practicing."

I don't think writing about this still untamed infection will somehow jinx me into death; I'm far too sophisticated for such paltry superstitions. On the other hand, if I do wind up dying of this thing, then perhaps I should have had more humility, plus respect, for the human urge to tap, count, or otherwise appease the gods. Should I expire imminently, I think I'd like written on my death certificate not *Staphylococcus*, but *Hubris*, perhaps as potent a poison as any. Or perhaps not. I don't know. I am not sure. To be on the safe side, tonight I'll bow my head in deference, say a prayer in pig Latin, count backwards from 100 in increments of seven, or do something equally unpleasant in order to demonstrate to the gods in my mind that I respect them despite my not believing in them. In the meantime, Dr. Shah's antibiotics will go to work in a far more logical fashion, knowing nothing of hubris or superstition or compulsions or plain old irrational fear. Each capsule autistic, its chemicals are incapable of knowing the nuance and needling of my mind. In this case, despite the fact that I too am a doctor—of psychology, that is—in this case, my mind is irrelevant, even if I can't say for sure that the gods are not.

Yes, that's what I said. A *doctor*. Of *psychology*. That I'm not a medical doctor but a mental doctor should make no difference at all, because anyone with an advanced degree of any sort should surely know by now that Descartes had it all wrong. The mind-body split has gone the way of espadrilles and iron lungs. In this day and age, we sophisticates understand that the division between the soul on one side and the skin on the other is mere illusion, a little trick our brain, with its putative "god nodules," plays on us. We further know that neurologists working at the forefront of illnesses like Parkinson's, which shares some features of—and has therefore galvanized some cures for—depression, are coming closer every day to a still clearer conviction that the physical suffering in our limbs and the mental suffering in our minds spurt from the same pool of chemicals in our own portable pharmaceutical factories. Now, it costs one heck of a lot to cryopreserve your entire self, but I once met a woman who was planning on freezing only her head after death. Her concern: "If they revive me, and reattach me to a body, and it's three thousand years later, won't I feel lonely in the world?" Heck yes. If you want to do something with your head once you're gone, give it to a brain bank. Let them slice you cold-cut thin, and hold your threaded meat up to brilliant lights and lenses. The answers to so many questions, and the cures for so much suffering, surely lie in that gray matter, which demands of its investigators a millimeter type of precision even as it suggests—in the story of its evolution from the Quarter Pounder it once was to the Big Mac it is today—some presence, or force—very fierce, yes—far too large for any test tube.

I got my doctorate in psychology in 1994. Specifically, my psychology degree is the lowly EdD, that scrappy acronym second best to the more regal and consonant PhD. The EdD doctorate—conferred upon one by a school of, of . . . *education*, that houses along with its would-be psychologists aspiring kindergarten teachers—is supposedly as crass and junky as a loud-mouthed woman wearing a chunky rock of a ring at a cocktail party for Brahmin intellectuals dressed in Brooks Brothers suits.

While I find absurd much of the jostling and hierarchical infighting of both academia and medicine, I have to admit that the EdD's status as a second-class citizen in the *Club des Docteurs* is not entirely undeserved. As an EdD, I am a bona fide doctor of some sort, but not once in graduate school did anyone require me to read any Freud. All right, all right, Freud is so *over*, but so is Latin, and learning it in high school did me a great deal of good. I can't speak for all EdD programs, or even for my EdD program; I can only speak about my experience in the program. It was as easy as easy could be. I learned to administer a lot of psychological tests, which allowed me to know the IQs of many close friends and also of my husband, who took his test stoned to the gills and still scored in the superior range. In graduate school, I actually had to study Carl Rogers and discuss for two semesters what it meant to hold patients in unconditional positive regard. Students learned how to "process," and anyone who confessed any type of subjective reaction during any class except statistics was seen as a sophisticate possessing insight. Thus there were many confessions that ranged from memories of mothers to bar mitzvah traumas to the deaths of all manner of minor pets. I was assigned not a single novel during my entire doctorate education, nor the tomes of a single theologist, many of whom have much to say about the human mind; on the other hand, I also was exposed to not one usable fact about biology, neurobiology, pathophysiology, or even the goddamn inner ear. It seems to me we students read mostly textbooks and discussed mostly transference, countertransference, and the administration of tests requiring write-ups so rote it would shock you to really know.

After graduation, I practiced as Dr. Slater for about twelve years. For the first year or two, the title "Doctor" seemed illicitly delicious, and I bought professional high heels and a savvy scarf to look the part. I loved my "patients." Although years have gone by now since I've stopped practicing, I still recall my patients' phone numbers, their medication dosages, their birthdays, their terrors, and their laughs, and their faces float through my dreams. I sometimes toy with the idea of calling one of my old patients up. It would be so good to hear the voice of someone I sat with two times a week for over a decade before I left the field. So good to check in, to find out more: babies, degrees, divorces? What stops me are the boundaries exerted by my guild, but even more, the sense that the call would, or might, satisfy only me.

The third thing that stops me is plain old fear. Unlike beautiful Dr. Shah and her pert prescription pad and the incredibly swift five-minute visit that yielded diagnosis, treatment plan, and pills in hand (pills, in this age of ever-mutating infections, with a still robust response rate), I sat with my patients through all sorts of wind and weather, snow and sleet, as time precipitated down around us, and gray moved to blue moved to bloom back into white again as winters came, and we all aged a decade or so together, and we all talked twenty thousand times more words than this essay contains, and my patients received more prescriptions from more pads than there are pages in this entire book, and yet they did not get better. They got company, which is what therapy is sure to give you (good or bad, no guarantee), but sanity, or just plain old peace of mind—no one really got that. I saw so much suffering. Let me tell you. No. No! I could not possibly even begin to tell you. So much suffering. So many souls tethered to so many brains brewing in so many cocktails of Clorazine and lithium and Effexor and Prozac and Zyprexa, each drug a dart in the dark, so the patients' brains in my mind are pocked and bubbled with blood where the darts of drugs have sunken. Some I loved. I want to call. But if they are dead, I do not want to know.

Throughout my years of practicing as a psychologist, I worked under several different supervisors, each, of course, with his or her own bias. I am quite sure medical doctors have their own biases as well, but in my opinion there is an immutability to medicine that puts natural parameters around bias and the extent to which it can go. I may be here inadvertently revealing my naïveté, but I'm not sure how much bias can affect the fact of clogged arteries, or, perhaps, of myocardial infarction, or even an infection and the microorganism responsible. I'm well aware that studies show how even the observer can change the observed, meaning pure objectivity is impossible. These sorts of studies and their postmodern implications fail to excite me. So *what* if 100 percent objectivity is beyond us? The 60 percent perfectly serviceable objectivity that comes with the practice of, say, vascular surgery, is pretty darn impressive to me, and it's enough, especially because I've never been too taken with perfection. Purity exits only in heaven, a place I have no interest in visiting any time soon.

For all *practical* intents and purposes, it seems to me (and if I'm wrong, darn it I'll feel dumb) that in the medical field, as well as in the bodies who seek its cures, gangrene is gangrene is gangrene and lupus is lupus is lupus. It further seems to me that in the field of mental health, no such solidity exists.

For instance, in my first three years practicing, substance abuse was very *in*, and while "codependency," "inner child," and all that other blather were never formal diagnostic terms, theorists like Alice Miller, whose work is saturated with such terms, and Bessel van der Kolk, who helped give "Trauma" its capital "T," ruled the day. Now, I have a great deal of respect for some of van der Kolk's work, a great deal less respect for the superficial ways he has been interpreted and the wholesale application of his theories to every other United States citizen, so that in the 1980s, the standard statistic was that one in three girls had been raped by a relative.

Given the era and its particular foci, in my first three years as a practicing psychologist, I was pressed to view almost every new patient as either a substance abuser or the traumatized child of a substance abuser whose inner child was beginning to "remember" some sort of sexual abuse that took place while one or the other was under the influence.

As someone who writes stories and believes narrative is sacred, I felt more than uncomfortable pressing preconceptions down upon people who had come for serious help for serious problems that deserved serious contemplation and the liminal state that almost always precedes conclusions with any integrity to them. We were rarely liminal. Thus, if I follow my own logic, we were often without integrity.

It hurts to hear that.

Hurts who?

Me. The one without.

In the practice of mental health treatment, diagnose someone as a substance abuser, and he or she will likely become one, not because the diagnosis necessarily causes the patient to drink more (although this is a possibility) but because the framework allows the practitioner to highlight that nightly crystal cup of merlot until the grapes glow ruby, and real.

This suggests many things, one of which is that narratives, despite their apparent binding in books, are in their true nature liquid and, once tossed into a man-made stream, will too easily conform to its contours, rushing over the rocks and echoing precisely the certain water-song that, in the instances I am speaking of, we psychologists wanted to hear.

A few years after I first entered the field as Dr. Slater, the man-made streambed shifted. Substance abuse as a primary diagnosis was on its way out; "dual diagnosis" was the big buzz word now, the general thought being that drug abuse was in reality a secondary problem; people abused drugs *because* they had a primary mood or anxiety disorder that often needed to be treated with licit drugs so they would no longer abuse illicit drugs. Now, this was quite the opposite of the salient ideas of just a few years earlier, when people's primary problem was their alcohol or drug abuse, both of which supposedly *caused* their mental health issues such as depression or anxiety. After all, most illicit drugs, and even the legal ones like alcohol, are either depressants or agitators. Therefore, in the years prior to the rise of dual diagnosis, what patients really needed to do was to cleanse their bodies of all drugs—licit, illicit, and anything in between. The shift, when it came, was seismic, and, like much tectonic activity, did little to clarify or construct.

Meanwhile Trauma and its offshoot, multiple personality disorder, continued to gain in popularity and there were more than a few times when I encountered would-be Sybils in my office, a phenomenon I had very little patience for, as it presented too many administrative hurdles and strained my "come on now" commonsense approach to the world. And then, eventually, multiple personality disorder was purged from the *Diagnostic and Statistical Manual* (DSM), the bible of mental health, a book which lists every kind of mental disorder under some men's short-lived suns, short-lived because the *Diagnostic Manual* is revised about every three years or so, sometimes even more frequently than that. In fact, in 2005 *The New Yorker* did a profile of the DSM's main architect, Dr. Robert Spitzer, who is so closely identified with his ever-morphing opus that a profile of Spitzer could not but be a profile of the DSM as well.

I enjoyed that profile for its sprightly writing, but I did not find it illuminating or surprising; it all felt quite familiar. After all, in the DSM-III-R, which was on the shelves when I first assumed the title of "Doctor," multiple personality disorder was in; in the DSM-IV diagnostic manual it was taken out, replaced by DID—dissociative identity disorder—which was so much less exciting to talk about that everyone stopped talking about it and, at least at my clinic, the diagnosis, once homecoming queen, went the way of the quiet kid in vocational school. I went from having six Sybils to none once MPD was eradicated and its popularity fell like the Dow on 9/11.

Premenstrual dysphoric disorder (PMDD) became a hot syndrome for a while when I was practicing, and lo and behold, I, who had never had a premenstrual problem in my life, suddenly started to realize that the two weeks before my period were far more hellish than the two weeks after my period. By now, almost ten years and three diagnostic manuals had gone by, and I was tiring of the ever-shifting streambed of categories and the illnesses they seemed to spur, but much more so of the a-reflective and zealous ways patients' stories got tossed in the air and patted like pizzas, stretched into whatever shape de jour was de jour. On top of that, the insurance industry was rapidly changing, expecting us to treat these ever-morphing syndromes—for which the synergy between the biological substrates and the cultural contexts seemed impossible to parse—in eight sessions or so. These factors, combined with the fact that I did not want to acquire PMDD, combined with the fact that I found scant fellowship amongst my colleagues, few of whom had the same questions and concerns about naming and shaping as did I, led me to quietly, without fanfare, leave the field, for what at first I called a small sabbatical, but for what has by now stretched into a solid seven years. Occasionally I contemplate going back, but this is always accompanied by a visceral sense of dread, of *defeat*, neither of which I feel when I imagine myself—writing income all dried up—being, say, a bike courier or a dog walker. I *mean* that. Thus, I stay away.

As for my periods—painless.

But things are never so simple. My leg is not so simple. Nor is it painless, despite Dr. Shah's impressively efficacious science, which has unfortunately, at this moment, bombed. Those oral antibiotics she prescribed, remember them? The autistic pills that could run my mind, with its little rituals, right into the ground—well, those capsule-sized quarterbacks seem to have gone on strike, but let me make one thing perfectly clear. As I said before: I don't believe belief has anything to do with this, although I'm sure if I read up on the potential power of a sugar pill, I might renege *somewhat* on my relatively unschooled opinion. We'll have to save that subject for another day, because on *this* day the drugs have failed, and as a result my leg is now hotter than hot and blazing with an aggressive infection no one knows how I could have acquired. Outside, late October, the fire department is preparing hydrants for winter by flushing them of their force; water tumbles into the streets, the sound of its pound and runnel everywhere. I smell rust in the warm autumn air.

Water is water is water. You can write it backwards as "Retaw" or splice it sideways so it reads "Taw/Re," but unlike all my Sybils, water will never change its properties in response to a human-made label; conversely, a human-made label will *never* create water. Cells, too, do not really respond to our descriptions of them; nor are they at all likely to alter their behavior or disappear should we cease to recognize them. There seems to me to be a certain solidity to the body and thus its human interventions that the mind and its doctors cannot lay claim to. Knowing this has hurt the pride of mental health practitioners, causing them to talk louder, longer, in ever more swirling spirals of jargon, as though that might be a bandage, some salve.

I don't mean to say the mind does not possess "real" measurable miseries with true biochemical substrates; it must, aplenty. The mind's miseries, however (at least, and perhaps if only, in light of our present-day biotechnological capacities), are invisible, test-tubed diseases, what cotton candy is to M&Ms, with their solid shells. Cotton candy melts away before you can quite clasp its fluff with your canines. This is mental illness, not necessarily in its essence but in our grasp, its manifestations morphing over the centuries in response to cultural pressures, fashions, and fads. To some degree, "physical" illness has done this too, but not nearly as much. Certainly no one would argue that environment affects the frequency with which we are stricken with conventional physical illnesses such as myocardia infarctions and high cholesterol, which I'm sure were far less common when we went naked and speared raw fish in oceans stocked with all variety of trout and tilapia, most now extinct, and likely before their time. However, unlike in the mental health field, diseases of the body are not, as far as I know, created and re-created every few years by a group of professors who sit around a table with coffee cups and Reubens and think up seemingly endless new shape sorters for the fog called human suffering and then slap some new improved name destined to design new improved symptoms, year after year after year. *The Diagnostic and Statistical Manual*, that bible brewed in mainly Manhattan, seems to have only a single fixed phenomenon, which is that for sure a revised edition will be created once the royalties on the current one run dry.

It is fascinating, and distressing, to look back at all the *Diagnostic and Statistical Manuals* since they first sprung into existence in 1952. The *DSM-I* has no use to the practitioner of today, for it describes illnesses no one has ever heard of, never mind figured out how to approach: "neurotic mood disorder" and "inward female masochism." Compare this to my husband's ancient medical tomes. While the cures have hugely progressed, the illnesses have for the most part stayed solid; blood vessels burst; microorganisms snack on fresh flesh; cells commit suicide; and eyes go badly blind. Gangrene and syphilis may be "gone" but their cousins are everywhere around, keeping up the family traditions. As my husband's tomes so surely show, since time immemorial the human heart has been vulnerable to cholesterol, but I doubt many cave men had ADHD, or even PTSD, though god knows they should have, what with all those mastodons running around.

It is for all these reasons that for me medicine has a certain stability and success. To some degree, to an impressive but incomplete degree, it has been able to locate the raw physical substrata of many human diseases, whereas in psychology and its allied fields, well, without a single simple blood test to tether us, we have fallen prey to a diagnostic drift that makes our pursuits seem somewhat pathetic, chintzy, when dressed up in the digs of science. And I dislike chintz, probably because I know I'm made of such material.

Beneath the fluff of our ever-morphing psychobabble, I think, or hope, there is a core called "soul," or even better, a penetrable and sensible series of syndromes that can either ultimately unify or finally separate everything from schizophrenia to dysthymia. But such unity, or separation, or even sense, is far harder to find in the brain than it is, say, in the leg, and all the hubbub and hysteria and jargon in the mental health field does little to help illuminate what is by all accounts an incredibly dense and challenging darkness the likes of which an ear doctor may never know. The dense darkness is real, as are the occasional pinpricks of light that allied fields like neurology give to the matter. The pinpricks of light, however, are not nearly enough to eradicate what are in truth, in the field of mental health, darts in the dark. So many darts in the dark. For this reason, a doctor of the body seems to me to be a true doctor; a doctor of the mind, a cotton candy chef.

Just before I quit psychology, my breast cells mutated en masse, right side, resulting, for me, in a bilateral mastectomy. I had understood the procedure as prophylactic—breast cancer runs in my family—but postsurgery, two different pathologists read into my smeared cells two very different stories. In story number one, I did indeed not have cancer, but rather cancer's precursor: *atypical ductal hyperplasia*. In story number two, however, created by a second pathololologist probably related somehow to my mother, who has never really approved of me, my breasts were loaded with *ductal carcinoma in situ*, otherwise known as cancer. *Cancer.* I read the words in my oncologist's chart before she could slap it shut. "I thought this was prophylactic," I said in my first post-op visit, still pale from the joint amputation. I lifted my hands to the two drains inserted into the hollowed cavities draining perpetual pus laced with threads of blood. The oncologist and I stared at each other. "I don't respect that second pathologist," she said, and then turned on her heel and left the room, holding my chart close to her own presumably intact breasts, as if to protect them, or maybe me.

I saw what she was trying to tell me. *Don't worry, Lauren.* But . . . but . . . this was *medicine*, for god's sake, not psychiatry. I learned a hard lesson that day. Medicine shed some of its Herculean heft as I found myself, like so many mental patients whose diagnoses change from year to year, swimming in a second narrative streambed packed with sharp rocks and deep drops into tidal pools in which lay a pale woman electrified by eelfish, a woman confused beneath a black and white sun, her pain intense but without name or even knowledge of its immortality, if that would have even helped her any, the foresight that her senseless suffering would be embalmed in a book that has survived the centuries, and tells us now, tonight, of times long long ago, when people not yet here were there.

From the could-be-breast-cancer confusion I was well reminded that even the sturdiest-seeming giants have gimp legs or athlete's foot or nits in their hair. I'm sure once I get really whacked with a truly hard-to-treat medical illness, I'll reexperience the real rock-'n'-roll Rorschach nature of traditional medicine with even more intensity, and maybe this time anger too. However, knowing that does not change the fact that if I had to choose between having schizophrenia and having multiple sclerosis, I'd rather have MS—not only because diseases that attack the mind attack the essence of who we are, while diseases that attack the flesh often can do no more than knock at the grand gates, but also because the MS clinics have clearer explanations and ever-more efficacious interventions for the sclerotic self than the Clozaril clinic does for all those schizophrenic selves who still, to this day, far too often, flail and wail away their days in some halfway house or on the streets of our cities in the cold dead of winter.

Dr. Slater. My schizophrenic patients used to call, used to wail, "Dr. Slater," tugging at their groins, their lips, fingers sunk to the knuckle in noses or ears. In the beginning, my illustrious title, as I said, levitated me; but by the end, let me tell you, it beat me back down to the ground, because I could offer no hard-core help for a syndrome, a disease, a devilish infiltration, a—*what? What?*
 What?

It may have happened after I lost a patient to suicide, or it could have occurred around the time my own psychopharmacologist explained to me that my ever-increasing and finally alarmingly large doses of Prozac had nothing to do with a phenomenon like tolerance and everything to do with the fact that *behind* the medicine my illness— sometimes depression, sometimes OCD, sometimes GAD, sometimes bipolar disorder—was doing push-ups, gaining in muscle and mass, training daily for its big breakthroughs. Those who work in the field of mental health have become masters at turning *the rational* into *a rationalization*. I would have far preferred it had my treating psychiatrist told me the truth: that he simply did not know why I had to keep increasing the dose of a medication supposedly immune to something like tolerance, just as we would never know why my patient, on the up and up, chose to put a bullet in one ear so it exited the other. In any case, the combination of failed interventions and rationalized cover-ups for what could have been real and regal question marks had a very physical effect on me, specifically on *my* ears. Eventually, whenever someone said the word "doctor" in reference to a psychiatrist or psychologist, no matter the speaker's nationality or region or religion, I started to always hear the title in a bothersome Texan twang and into my mind popped up not the image of a doctor but of a stewardess in pink lipstick. I know the stewardess piece makes little sense, but who cares. I hate to fly; thus the image was doubly unpleasant.

Inevitably, the Texan twang moved inside of me so when I said to myself, "Dr. Slater," I heard in my title a farce, a taunt. I heard my title all wrong, because I'm not from Texas but from Boston. After some months of this, the wrongness went from odd to ominous and the very word itself—"docteurrr"—headed across the ocean, to Germany, where it took up a Teutonic hum reminiscent of B-grade Nazi movies. It must have been at least a year before the simple bisyllabic utterance of "doctor" shed its limbic melodrama and peregrinate ways and settled down in a higher, drier, saner spot in my head, allowing me to view the problem primarily as grammatical. Was I a noun or a verb? A doctor is a noun, but *to* doctor is a verb. In general I prefer verbs to nouns, but this was an exception. I was a verb wanting to be a noun, and knowing it would not happen. *To doctor:* to change or alter dishonestly. To cover up. To fake.

So this is not, in the end, a story about becoming a doctor, but about un-becoming a doctor, or de-doctoring this doctor. And what was beneath? What have we here? A middle-aged woman with a cat and a dog who knows that schizophrenia is 295.20 in the newest *Diagnostic and Statistical Manual* (until next year, when something is added or subtracted in a revision that reflects the writing of a novel far more than the testing of a hypothesis), but beyond that, who knows not much more about the human psyche than any kind, insightful soul with good ears and a good heart, cholesterol-clogged or not.

As for my husband's medical books, they tell a story far denser than what my children grasp. The gangrene girl of the eighteenth century eventually morphs, ten dusty volumes later, into Jonas Salk and the discovery of antibiotics so effective we have almost wrung them dry. In fact, as it turns out, Dr. Shah's first prescription has not worked—not worked!—and the infection is dancing down my body in dark red streams.

My husband drives me to the hospital in a drizzle as fine and sticky as hairspray, and for two days I lie on a narrow bed mainlining whatever they've got to give me while considering what it might be like to lose my leg. The doctor's helplessness, however, stems not from lack of knowledge but from the increasingly frequent failure of overused antibiotics. Thus our newest "superbugs," which word brings to my mind a TWA-sized insect flying in a Crayola blue sky. I lie tethered to my hospital IV and, in a fever, converse with this insect, born, he tells me, from the forehead of a forefather who will take my leg once it is completely claimed by beetles.

I once had a patient named Pepsi, a tiny Vietnamese man who spoke at best broken English and who cut off his own testicle because the voice of Mother Mary told him to. Once that body part was gone, Pepsi went for another, and another, and another, until, a decade later, his hand was a mere mitt missing all its fingers, the seamed scars shiny, his touch spastic and bony. We could not stop Pepsi's infection, whatever it was, and instead of grieving that, we sat in meetings and dissected the diagnoses, hip-hopping back and forth between mania and schizophrenia, lithium and Clozaril, neither one making a difference. We never truly admitted that. *Didn't make a difference.* It hurt too much to say that. We didn't want to lose our own limbs in the process. Pepsi, where are you now, my little man? I remember you.

I don't remember, however, how many days it really was before the red spread of my own infection finally paused, reflected, and then decided to retreat, defeated or maybe just plain bored. The strangest thing is, I saw it go. The doctors had my leg hiked high in the air and I saw the infection stall, and then heard the thrum of its Army Hummers as they all at once thrust into reverse and backed out, so that bit by bit my leg's peach complexion returned. Thus on a gorgeous October day—the leaves so fevered my daughter caught their heat and exclaimed, "Autumn is the season when all the trees have a beautiful disease"—I was discharged from the hospital, with a new plan, and new pills in hand.

Twice a day now I swallow my mighty Bactrin and its ancillary troops, and moment-by-moment my leg reclaims its color. Thank you doctor, Baily. Thank you doctor, Shah. I would say you are worthy of your titles. That I am not worthy of mine saddens me not a bit. Don't call me Dr. Slater. Call me who I am. My name is Lauren, and if your soul is sick, you can come to visit me. Even though there is not yet, and maybe never will be, a simple single pill or silver scalpel for your suffering, that doesn't mean I don't have a very dignified job to do. It's called "keeping company." It's called "imparting hope." It's called "mopping up grief and changing the bedpan when it's full of too many tears and tissues." That, in truth, is what real "doctors" called psychologists often do, and once you put down your plastic stethoscope and your bottle of candied pills, the quiet dignity of hard human work returns, and you remember that while "real" flesh-based medicine has amazing capacities to heal, not all doctors in those ever-fragmenting medical fields have retained the capacity to hear the suffering beneath the syndromes they have the know-how to treat. And if psychology's great crime is claiming for itself a scientific method it has no real right to, medicine's great crime is churning out human doctors who know only craft, not kindness, and thus have lost their humanity, having forgotten, as scientists, how to pay homage to mystery. To humility. To superstition. Yes, superstition.

Knock knock. Who's there? Lauren. Lauren who? Lauren Slater, a name with nothing in front, and nothing in back, just two proper nouns that sit so small on this page. Now there's a fact—*so small, my name*—something I can measure, something I can count, like the pages in my husband's dusty tomes. In my mending, I, like my children, drag the tomes to bed, flip through centuries and scalpels until at last sleep snows me down, so I barely hear the thud as the volume hits the floor and shatters, like glass, into glinting bits everywhere on the bedroom floor. As I reach to pick up the million pieces, a voice says, *This is just a dream,* and yet it seems so real. Once, dreams were serious symbols. Most psychologists today would suggest dreams symbolize nothing; rather they merely reflect the chaos of our p.m. chemicals. I don't know, as I am not—knock knock—Dr. Slater anymore. I am, instead, reaching for this broken book. Leaning from my sickbed, I scoop some stories up, and as I do, a shard slices me sideways and my hand begins to bleed. Infection! Infection! *It's just a dream.* But I can't come out, and yet, suddenly, I am no longer scared. I always wondered what would kill me and now, finally, I know. That there is much I don't know is okay. I watch my hand empty out, all the platelets and cells so visible it's like a science exhibit about platelets and cells, and the blood isn't red this time. It is, or maybe I am, a true teal, and it just keeps coming, I just keep coming, on and on, an actual color, a pulse; profusely.

CONTRIBUTOR NOTes

CHARLES BARDES lives and practices in New York City, where he is Professor of Clinical Medicine and Associate Dean at Weill Cornell Medical College. "The Doctor in Middle Age" is excerpted from his manuscript *The Double Serpent: Subtexts in Medicine*, selections of which also appear in the print and online versions of the journal *AGNI*. His most recent book, *Pale Faces: The Masks of Anemia* (Bellevue Literary Press, 2008), investigates the cultural, literary, and mythological associations of a common disease construct.

MARION BISHOP earned a PhD in English and American Literature from New York University and an MD from the University of Utah. She lives in northern Utah and works as an ER doctor in rural Wyoming.

ROBERT COLES is the recipient of numerous awards, including a Pulitzer Prize for General Non-Fiction in 1973 for his series of books *Chil-*

dren of Crisis; a MacArthur Award in 1981; the Presidential Medal of Freedom in 1998; and the National Humanities Medal in 2001. He has written more than seventy-five books and writes regular columns for *The New Republic, New Oxford Review,* and *American Poetry Review.*

SAYANTANI DASGUPTA is a writer, physician, and medical humanities educator. She is an Assistant Professor of Clinical Pediatrics and core faculty in the Program in Narrative Medicine at Columbia University. She also teaches courses in illness narratives and narrative genetics at Sarah Lawrence College, where she is a prose faculty member in the summer "Writing the Medical Experience" conference. She is the co-author of *The Demon Slayers and Other Stories: Bengali Folktales,* the author of a memoir about her time at Johns Hopkins Medical School, *Her Own Medicine: A Woman's Journey from Student to Doctor*; and the co-editor of a book of women's illness narratives, *Stories of Illness and Healing: Women Write Their Bodies.* DasGupta is an associate editor of the journal *Literature and Medicine,* and an editorial board member of the online journal *Pulse.* She also publishes personal essays, creative nonfiction, and academic articles on the role of narrative in medicine. She is particularly interested in exploring storied approaches to health care and social justice. However, DasGupta's most important stories are lived in the context of her family—as a daughter, spouse, and mother to her two young children.

ELISSA ELY is a graduate of Harvard Medical School. She completed her residency in Community Psychiatry, worked many years in a Massachusetts state hospital, and now works in an outpatient clinic for the U.S. Department of Mental Health, as well as several Boston area shelters.

THOMAS C. GIBBS is a practicing obstetrician-gynecologist in Orlando, Florida. He has published poems, essays, and articles in the *Yale Journal for Humanities and Medicine, Stone Canoe, The Healing Muse, Hospital Drive,* and *The Sylvan Echo.*

KAY REDFIELD JAMISON is Professor of Psychiatry at the Johns Hopkins University School of Medicine and Co-Director of the Johns Hopkins Mood Disorders Center. She is also Honorary Professor of English at the University of St. Andrews. She is the co-author of the standard medical text *Manic-Depressive Illness: Bipolar Disorders and Recurrent Depression,* as well as author of *An Unquiet Mind; Night Falls Fast: Understanding Suicide; Touched with Fire: Manic-Depressive Illness and the Artistic Temperament; Exuberance: The Passion for Life;* and *Nothing Was the Same: A Memoir.* She is a John D. and Catherine T. MacArthur Fellow.

SANDEEP JAUHAR is a cardiologist and director of the Heart Failure Program at Long Island Jewish Medical Center. He writes regularly for the *New York Times* and the *New England Journal of Medicine,* and his first book, *Intern,* was published in early 2008 by Farrar, Straus & Giroux. He lives with his wife, Sonia, and their children, Mohan and Pia, in New York City.

PERRI KLASS is the author of books, essays, award-winning short stories, a novel, and numerous articles ranging from professional papers to popular journalism and travel pieces. Her 1987 book, *A Not Entirely Benign Procedure,* chronicled her medical school years; her 2007 book, *Treatment Kind and Fair: Letters to a Young Doctor,* looked at changes in medicine and medical education. Her most recent book is *The Mercy Rule*, a novel. She is a professor of journalism and pediatrics at New York University, and she writes the "18 and Under" column for the *New York Times*.

PETER D. KRAMER is an American psychiatrist, former Marshall Scholar, and faculty member of Brown Medical School specializing in the area of depression. Kramer is the author of six books, including a novel, *Spectacular Happiness* (2001), and the international bestseller *Listening to Prozac* (1993), a work that worries over the possibility of "cosmetic psychopharmacology"—a term Kramer coined to describe the use of medication to tweak personality traits.

LEAH E. MINTZ graduated Phi Beta Kappa and Magna cum Laude from the University of California, Los Angeles before receiving her medical degree at the UCLA School of Medicine. She completed her residency training in otolaryngology–head and neck surgery at the UCLA School of Medicine in June 2000. Dr. Mintz is a diplomat of the American Board of Otolaryngology and a member of both the Los Angeles Society and the American Academy of Otolaryngology–Head and Neck Surgery. She is published in the fields of head and neck cancer and immunotherapy, and has presented her work at the national meetings of the American Academy of Otolaryngology–Head and Neck Surgery and the American Head and Neck Society.

CLINT MOREHEAD received his undergraduate degree from Bellarmine University in 2004 and his MD from the University of Louisville in 2008. He is currently a first-year internal medicine resident at the University of Louisville. In 2007, he founded the Kentucky Books for Patients Project, an organization that places books by Kentucky authors in cancer centers across the state.

DANIELLE OFRI is a physician at Bellevue Hospital in New York City. She is best known for *Singular Intimacies: Becoming a Doctor at Bellevue*, the classic story of becoming a doctor by immersion at the oldest public hospital in the country—and perhaps the most legendary. Ofri is also editor-in-chief of the *Bellevue Literary Review*, the first literary journal to arise from a medical center.

TERI REYNOLDS received her doctorate in literature from Columbia University and her medical degree from the University of California, San Francisco. She practices as an emergency physician in Oakland and San Francisco, where she lives with her husband and son.

PEGGY SARJEANT lives in Seattle, Washington, with her husband, two teenagers, two 110-pound Bernese mountain dogs, and a cat that rules the world. Her short fiction has appeared in the *Portland Review* and in *Cutthroat, A Journal of the Arts*. One of her stories was awarded third prize by the Pacific Northwest Writers' Association in their 2008 Short Fiction Contest, and another was the recipient of the 2008 Albert and Elaine Borchard Fellowship for Fiction at the Tomales Bay Writers' Workshops. She recently completed her first collection of short fiction. Peggy practiced General Pediatrics for eighteen years. She dedicates this essay to Marilyn Guthrie.

LAUREN SLATER is a psychologist and the author of *Opening Skinner's Box: Great Psychological Experiments of the Twentieth Century*; *Welcome to My Country*; and *Lying: A Metaphorical Memoir*. She has been the recipient of numerous awards, including a 2004 National Endowment for the Arts Award and a Knight Science Journalism Fellowship at the Massachusetts Institute of Technology. Slater is a contributing writer to *Elle* magazine, has had multiple appearances in *Best American* volumes, and is a frequent contributor to the *New York Times Magazine*, in Somerville, Mas-

School in 1986. He cur- fornia, working a three- day-on (twelve-hour shifts), medically themed novel, *Death on the East Annex* (Silverleaf Press), will be published in the fall of 2010. He lives in Laguna Beach with his wife and three dogs.

ZALDY S. TAN is Director of Education at the Brigham and Women's Hospital Division of Aging and Assistant Professor of Medicine at Harvard Medical School.

ABIGAIL ZUGER is a physician in New York City and a frequent contributor of essays, reviews, and articles to both medical and lay publications, including the *New England Journal of Medicine* and the science section of the *New York Times*. Her book about the early days of AIDS, *Strong Shadows: Scenes from an Inner City AIDS Clinic*, was published by W. H. Freeman & Co. in 1995.